Female Reproductive Health

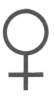

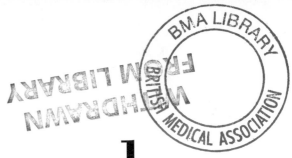

Female Reproductive Health

Edited by

Nikolai Manassiev
The Wand Medical Centre
Birmingham, UK

and

Malcolm I. Whitehead
King's College Hospital
London, UK

The Parthenon Publishing Group
International Publishers in Medicine, Science & Technology

A CRC PRESS COMPANY
BOCA RATON   LONDON   NEW YORK   WASHINGTON, D.C.

Library of Congress Cataloging-in-Publication Data

Female reproductive health/edited by Nikolai Manassiev, Malcolm Whitehead.

   p. ; cm

Includes bibliographical references and index.

ISBN 1–85070–491–0 (alk. paper)

   1. Gynecology. 2. Reproductive health. 3. Women–Health and hygiene. I. Manassiev, Nikolai. II. Whitehead, Malcolm I.

   [DNLM: 1. Reproduction-physiology. 2. Genital Diseases, Female. 3. Genitalia, Female-physiology. 4. Infection. WQ 205 F3287 2003]

RG 133. F45 2003

618.1-dc21   2003045973

British Library Cataloguing in Publication Data

Female reproductive health

   1. Gynecology 2. Generative organs, Female

   I. Manassiev, Nikolai II. Whitehead, Malcolm I.

   618.1

ISBN 1-85070-491-0

Published in the USA by
The Parthenon Publishing Group
345 Park Avenue South, 10th Floor
New York, NY 10010, USA

Published in the UK and Europe by
The Parthenon Publishing Group
23–25 Blades Court
Deodar Road
London SW15 2NU, UK

Copyright © 2004
The Parthenon Publishing Group

Typeset by Siva Math Setters, Chennai, India
Printed and bound by Antony Rowe Ltd., Chippenham, Wiltshire, UK

Contents

List of contributors

Naim Abusheikha
Bourn Hall Clinic
Cambridge CB3 7TR
UK

Henry Burger
Prince Henry's Institute of Medical Research
Monash Medical Centre
Clayton
Victoria
Australia

John Collins
Department of Obstetrics and Gynecology
McMaster University
Hamilton
Ontario L8N 3Z5
Canada

Fergus Keating
Giggs Hill Surgery
14 Raphael Drive
Thames Ditton
Surrey KT7 OEB
UK

Joanna N. Raeburn
King's College Hospital NHS Trust
Denmark Hill
London SE5 9Rs
UK

Alison Stirland
Sexually Transmitted Disease Program
Los Angeles Department of Health
Los Angeles
CA 90007
USA

Chris Wilkinson
Margaret Pyke Centre and Camden &
Islington Contraceptive and Reproductive
Health Services
73 Charlotte Street
London WIT 4PL
UK

The female reproductive system – anatomy and physiology

1

Nikolai Manassiev and Fergus Keating

INTRODUCTION

The female reproductive system is composed of the internal and external genitalia. The internal genitalia comprise the ovaries, uterine (fallopian) tubes, uterus (including the cervix) and vagina. The external genitalia consist of the vulva, which comprises the labia majora, labia minora, clitoris, vestibular bulbs, mons veneris (pubis), urethral and peri-urethral gland ducts. The vulva serves as the entrance to the vagina and in the normal state covers and protects the urethral orifice.

The breast is not essential for reproduction. However, it poses a constant challenge with early cancer detection and it brings misery to many women in the form of pain. So it is essential that the breast should be included in this discussion.

EXTERNAL GENITALIA

Labia majora

These are two skin folds overlying a condensation of fat, connective and elastic tissue and muscle fibers (Figure 1.1). These folds continue cranially toward the lower abdomen and fuse in the midline as the anterior commissure, or the mons pubis. The caudal union of the labia is known as the posterior commissure. The outer borders of the labia majora define the lateral extent of the vulva. The skin covering the labia majora is thick, contains many sebaceous and sweat glands and is covered with hair, except along the lower part of the inner aspect. The skin is composed of stratified squamous epithelium with a well-vascularized dermis. The round ligaments that emerge from the inguinal canal enter the labia in the upper third.

Labia minora

The labia minora consist of two cutaneous folds, which are usually concealed by the labia majora (Figure 1.1). They directly approximate each other, thus covering the vaginal opening. The labia minora extend from the clitoris anteriorly to the posterior fourchette, where they join the labia majora. Sweat glands and follicles are usually absent, but sebaceous glands are abundant. The epithelium is stratified and squamous, with minimal keratinization. The prepuce of the clitoris is continuous with the labia minora and is histologically similar, except for its extreme vascularity. Usually the mons and the labia majora are the only visible parts of the external genitals. The labia minora are in contact with each other thus closing the vaginal opening. The space bounded by the labia minora and the vaginal opening is called vestibule. The latter forms a junction between the external and internal genitals. In this space are the openings of the urethra, vagina and the greater vestibular glands (Bartholin's glands). The Bartholin's glands secrete a milky lubricant during sexual arousal. Minor vestibular glands secrete mucus around the clitoris and the urethral orifice. The vestibular fossa is the tissue between the vaginal opening and posterior fourchette. The vestibule has two spongy bulbs, one on each side. These bulbs are erectile and meet in the middle thus resembling a horseshoe from an anterior position. During sexual stimulation

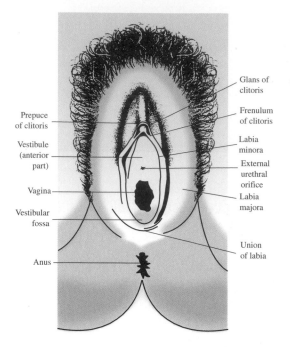

Prepuce of clitoris

Vestibule (anterior part)

Vagina

Vestibular fossa

Anus

Glans of clitoris

Frenulum of clitoris

Labia minora

External urethral orifice

Labia majora

Union of labia

Figure 1.1 Components of the vulva. Reproduced from Romanes GJ. *Cunningham's Manual of Practical Anatomy*, 14th edn. Vol. 11, Thorax and Abdomen. Oxford: Oxford University Press, 1977:169, reproduced with permission of Oxford University Press

they become engorged. For further discussion about the role of the vestibule in sexual dysfunction, see Chapter 9, page 178.

Clitoris

The clitoris is composed of two roots that run along the lower pubic rami to unite beneath the symphysis in the body of the clitoris. The distal part of the body is the glans. The ischiocavernosus muscle covers the root and the body of the clitoris. The roots, or crura, are 3–4 cm long in the flaccid state, but when erect are 4.5–5 cm long. The body is 2.3–3 cm long and is surrounded by a connective tissue fascia. The covering of the glans is modified cutaneous tissue and not mucosa. Unlike the penis, the glans clitoris contains no corpus spongiosum and does not possess as much erectile tissue. There are numerous sensory nerve endings for touch and pressure, such as Meissner's corpuscles, on the clitoris. This

little organ has 8000 nerve fibers – double that of the penis. The sensory supply is via the pudendal nerve. There is also sympathetic innervation via the pelvic sympathetic plexuses.

The clitoris seems to function as the nerve center for coitus. Sexual stimulation causes vascular engorgement and enlargement. This makes the clitoris exquisitely sensitive to the friction of the inserted penis. Orgasm in the female consists of a reflex resulting in forceful contractions of both voluntary and involuntary muscles of the pelvis and pelvic viscera. It may result from stimulation of the clitoris even in the absence of the vagina. Once the process of orgasm has been experienced and a conditional reflex has been established, then the presence of the clitoris is no longer essential for orgasm. It is said that women who have undergone vulvectomy with excision of the clitoris are still capable of experiencing orgasm.

The arterial supply to the vulva is mainly via the internal pudendal artery. The veins approximate the same course but also communicate with the vesicovaginal plexus and the inferior hemorrhoidal veins. The lymph drains via the inguinal and femoral nodes to the external iliac nodes. The nerve supply is from multiple sources. The main contributor is the pudendal nerve, which is derived from the second to fourth sacral nerves: the ilioinguinal and the genitofemoral nerves also contribute.

INTERNAL GENITALIA

Vagina

The vagina is a musculomembranous canal extending from the vulva to the uterine cervix (Figures 1.2–1.3). It is directed upward and posteriorly from the vestibule toward the sacral promontory. Anteriorly, the vagina is closely related to the bladder and urethra. The urethra lies against the lower two-thirds of the vagina and the bladder trigone against the upper third. The tissues separating these structures are called the urethrovaginal and

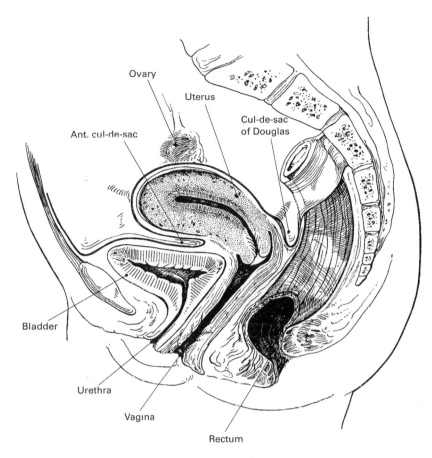

Figure 1.2 Sagittal section of the human female pelvis. Reproduced with permission from Bengtson J. The vagina and female urology. In Ryan KJ, Friedman AJ, Barbieri RL, eds. *Kistner's Gynecology*, 5th edn. Chicago: Year Book Medical Publishing, 1990:112

vesicovaginal septa, respectively, and consist of supporting tissues of the endopelvic fascia. The posterior vaginal wall is related to the peritoneal cul-de-sac (pouch of Douglas) in its upper third, to the ampulla of the rectum in its middle third, and to the perineal body in its lower third. The perineal body is an important structure that provides a central area of insertion of the supporting muscles of the pelvic floor. At the introitus, the vagina is related laterally to the bulbocavernous muscles. Superiorly, the upper vagina fuses with the cervix, which projects into it through its anterior wall. As a result of this arrangement, the posterior wall of the vagina is longer than the anterior wall by about 2–3 cm. The recesses of the vaginal vault above the cervix are called fornices,

the deepest being the posterior fornix. The vaginal length is usually 8–10 cm. The perineal muscles cause relative constriction of the outlet diameter. The vagina is flattened when relaxed, creating only potential space, but has a remarkable ability to distend, for example, during the process of delivery, to accommodate the passage of the fetus. The vaginal wall possesses multiple circumferential folds, or rugae. The folds become less prominent after the menopause. The vaginal lining is often referred to as vaginal skin and this term is useful in everyday practice. Histologically, however, the vagina has three layers: mucous membrane, muscular layer and adventitia. The mucosa is composed of a non-keratinized squamous epithelium. The epithelium is

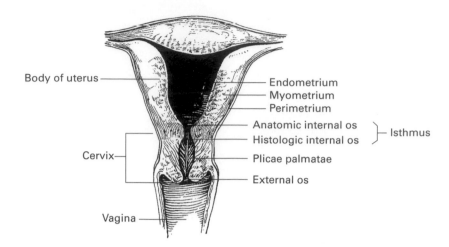

Figure 1.3 Frontal section of the uterine cervix and corpus. Reproduced with permission from Sheets EE, Goodman HM, Knapp RC. The cervix. In Ryan KJ, Friedman AJ, Barbieri RL, eds. *Kistner's Gynecology*, 5th edn. Chicago: Year Book Medical Publishing, 1990:146

continuous onto the vaginal portion of the cervix. Vaginal epithelial cells contain abundant glycogen, especially at midcycle, when plasma estradiol levels are high. The vagina is well vascularized but does not contain glands. During sexual excitement, the blood vessels engorge, the vaginal skin reddens and a transudate is released into the vagina to aid lubrication.

The vaginal epithelium undergoes changes under the influence of estrogen. Estrogen induces proliferation and maturation of the epithelium, enhances glycogen storage in the superficial cells and increases the blood flow to the paravaginal tissues. This leads to increased epithelial thickness and strengthening of the mechanical barrier between the vagina and the outside environment.

There are three cell types present in the vaginal epithelium: parabasal cells, the intermediate cell layer and superficial cells. Under the influence of estrogen the superficial cells predominate during the reproduction years, while in estrogen deprivation, i.e., after the menopause, there is a predominance of parabasal and intermediate cells. The normal vaginal pH is 3.5–4.5 and this acidity is due to conversion of the glycogen stored in the superficial and intermediate cells into lactic acid by lactobacilli. The normal vaginal flora and physiology is discussed in more detail in Chapter 7.

The vaginal blood supply is from the internal pudendal artery, a branch of the internal iliac artery with wide anastomoses with the uterine, inferior vesical and middle rectal vessels. The lymph from the upper two-thirds drains into the external and internal iliac nodes, while that from the lower third drains into the inguinal nodes. The sensory innervation of the vagina is from the pudendal and ilioinguinal nerves. Sympathetic fibers from the hypogastric plexuses supply blood vessels and the smooth muscle of the vaginal wall. The upper vagina is said to be sensitive only to stretching.

Uterus and fallopian tubes

The uterus (Figures 1.2–1.4) consists of two parts: the uterine cervix and uterine body. The cervix is cylindrical and points downward and backward. It measures 2.5–3 cm in length and 2–3 cm in diameter in adult nulligravid women, but its size can vary considerably between women. The cervix is connected to the uterine body by the isthmus. The vagina attaches to the cervix around its middle (length) and divides the cervix into vaginal and supravaginal parts. In the center of the vaginal part of the cervix there is a small opening – the external os – by which the cavity of the uterus communicates with the vagina. The cervical canal extends from the external os to the anatomic internal os, where it connects with the uterine cavity. The cervical canal is spindle-shaped, measuring about 8 mm at its greatest width. The isthmus is the area of the uterus that lies between the anatomic internal os above and the histologic internal os below. The latter represents the area of transition from endometrial to endocervical glands. The isthmus is referred to as the lower uterine segment during pregnancy and labor.

The cervix secretes mucus which is subject to cyclical changes. Following menses, the amount of mucus secreted by the endocervical glands is reduced and it is viscous. The quantity of mucus increases up to 30-fold in response to increasing levels of estrogens during the second half of the follicular phase. The mucus becomes thin, watery, clear and elastic and is then highly permeable to spermatozoa. A fine thread of mucus (up to 10 cm long) can be demonstrated by stretching a drop of secretion (spinnbarkeit) on a microscope slide. A characteristic ferning, or palm leaf arborization, can be seen if mucus is dried on a slide. During the luteal phase and during pregnancy, the mucus acts as a plug between the uterus and the external environment. Progesterone secretion during the luteal phase makes the mucus thick, milky white and a barrier for sperm and possibly microorganisms.

The cervix is covered by two different types of epithelium: squamous and columnar. The area of the cervix where the stratified squamous epithelium of the vagina becomes the columnar epithelium of the endocervix is known as the transformation zone. The position of the transformation zone is related to age, age at first pregnancy and the degree of estrogenic stimulation. During the reproductive years, the endocervical epithelium and glands extend to the level of the external os or just above it. Under estrogenic stimulation, such as that resulting from the oral contraceptive pill or from pregnancy, the endocervical epithelium may migrate beyond the external os, appearing as a visible area on the cervix that was known, misleadingly, as a cervical erosion – misleading, as it incorrectly

implies a pathologic change. The proper term for this condition is cervical eversion/ectropion. During the latter half of fetal life a similar proliferation of the endocervical mucosa may occur which can produce a congenital eversion seen in up to 50% of female neonates. After the menopause, as a result of waning ovarian activity, the endocervical mucosa retracts upward and the transformation zone (squamocolumnar junction) can disappear from view. If this occurs then obtaining a cervical smear or performing colposcopy may not be possible unless estrogenic stimulation is applied for several weeks beforehand. The cervical eversion (ectropion) can spontaneously disappear and the squamocolumnar junction can move above the external os during the reproductive years as well. This process is known as squamous metaplasia.

Squamous metaplasia

Metaplasia implies transformation of one type of differentiated tissue into another. In the cervix, squamous metaplasia occurs when the prolapsed endocervical epithelium (eversion/ectropion) is replaced by the more robust squamous epithelium. The process of metaplasia probably involves the following steps:

(1) Endocervical eversion, metaplasia and stratification of the cell layer which is underneath the eversion;

(2) Sloughing of the overlying columnar epithelium;

(3) Maturation of the underlying cells into stratified squamous epithelium.

The mature metaplastic epithelium is indistinguishable from the indigenous squamous epithelium. However, the immature metaplastic epithelium lacks glycogen and does not take up iodine, which can confuse the inexperienced colposcopist. The presence of metaplastic cells on a cervical smear is thus a normal finding.

The body of the uterus measures 7–7.5 cm in length, 4.5–5 cm in width and 2.5–3 cm in

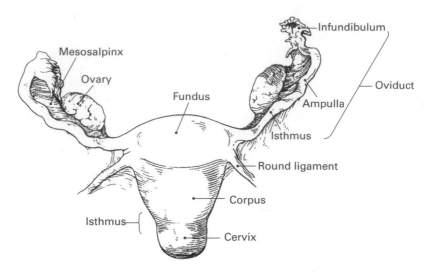

Figure 1.4 Anterior view of the uterus. Reproduced with permission from Fincker NJ, Friedman AJ. The uterine corpus. In Ryan KJ, Friedman AJ, Barbieri RL. *Kistner's Gynecology*, 5th edn. Chicago: Year Book Medical Publishing, 1990:189

thickness. It lies in the pelvis between the bladder and the rectum. The cephalic portion is called the fundus. On both sides of the fundus are the uterine horns where the fallopian tubes join the uterus. The uterus is composed mainly of smooth muscle cells wrapped in peritoneum on the outside. On the inside of the uterus there is a cavity lined with endometrium. It is slit-like and triangular in shape. The uterus has a remarkable potential to grow. It can grow from 50–100 g in the non-pregnant state to over 1 kg during pregnancy. The uterine endometrium also changes under the influence of ovarian hormones, developing from less than 5 mm in thickness during the early follicular phase and in menopausal women, to more than 10 mm under the influence of estrogen.

The fallopian tubes connect the ovaries with the uterus (Figure 1.4). They are about 10–12 cm in length. Their reproductive function involves ovum collection and transport, the transport of sperm, aiding fertilization and early embryonic development, and transport of the conceptus to the uterus. The fallopian tubes are under the influence of ovarian hormones: their motility changes as the viscosity of the tubal fluid and the ciliary action of mucosal cells change cyclically.

The blood supply to the uterus and the tubes is by the uterine artery, a branch of the internal ileac artery. The venous blood drains to the internal ileac veins and there are extensive communications with the vesical and rectal plexuses. The main lymphatic drainage is to the external and internal iliac nodes and there are some scanty connections to the inguinal and aortic nodes. The nerves to the uterus and tubes are branches from the pelvic plexus. Pain from the cervix is carried by pelvic splanchnic nerves (parasympathetic), while that from the body of the uterus (labor pains) travels with sympathetic fibers to the lowest thoracic segments of the cord – T11–T12. The abolition of all uterine sensation requires destruction/anesthesia above the T10 level.

Ovary

The two ovaries (Figure 1.4) are almond-shaped organs 2–5 cm in length, 1.5–3 cm wide and 0.5–1.5 cm thick. The combined weight is about 15–20 g. Each is suspended to the uterus via the uteroovarian ligament and to the fallopian tube via the infundibulopelvic ligament. When the woman is standing, the long axis of the ovary is vertical and its lateral surface lies against the pelvic side wall. The ovary is attached to the posterior leaf of the broad ligament by a peritoneal fold termed the mesovarium. It derives its blood supply from the ovarian artery, a branch of the abdominal aorta just below the renal artery. The venous drainage parallels the artery and the lymphatics drain to the para-aortic nodes, just above the level of the umbilicus (L3/L4).

The ovary has a complex structure and function, being an organ of gametogenesis and also an endocrine organ. It consists of three distinct regions: the outer cortex, which contains the ovarian follicles, a central medulla consisting of ovarian stroma, and an inner hilum around the area of attachment of the ovary to the mesovarium. The development of the ovary involves three distinct embryonic tissues: the primordial germ cells, the coelomic epithelium of the urogenital ridge, and the ovarian mesenchyme. The primordial germ cells originate from the gut endoderm and give rise to the oocytes, the granulosa cells develop from the coelomic epithelium and the stromal and thecal cells arise from the mesenchyme. The ovary develops from the genital ridge, which starts to form from about the fifth to sixth week of fetal development. It consists of an inner core of ovarian mesenchyme and a thick outer layer of proliferating coelomic epithelium. At this stage, male and female gonads are indistinguishable and are known as indifferent gonads ('indifferent' is the correct embryologic term). In the absence of the Y chromosome, the indifferent gonad develops into an ovary. The germ cells develop from the yolk sac and migrate and settle in the ovary, as oogonia. They proliferate through mitosis until about 20 to 38 weeks' gestation when mitotic division ceases and meiosis starts. The oogonia differentiate into primary oocytes, which progress into the prophase of the first meiotic division and then become dormant until puberty. In other words, at the time of her birth, a female has all the oocytes she will ever have. At 25–28 weeks of gestation, the number of oocytes peaks at around six to seven million and then their number starts a steady decline, the loss

being due to atresia. At birth, there are approximately one million germ cells, and at the time of puberty, there are between 250 000 and 400 000 oocytes. After puberty, in the oocytes that are destined for ovulation, following the preovulatory luteinizing hormone (LH) surge, meiosis is resumed and the first division is completed with the formation of a big daughter cell and the extrusion of the small polar body. The oocyte enters the second meiotic division and is arrested in its metaphase (metaphase II). Resumption of the second meiotic division follows sperm fusion, resulting in the formation of a second polar body and female pronucleus.

Follicles

The follicles are situated in the ovarian cortex and are either dormant or in various stages of development (Figure 1.5). The inactive follicles are termed primordial. In each cycle, a cohort of primordial follicles is recruited and starts developing. The primordial follicle is composed of a single layer of granulosa cells and a single immature oocyte arrested in the first meiotic division. The follicle is separated from the surrounding stroma by a thin basement membrane and does not have a direct blood supply. The developing primordial follicles go through the following stages: primary, secondary, tertiary, graafian and atretic. The first three stages of growth can occur in the absence of gonadotropins and thus suggest either intraovarian control or pre-programed recruitment. During these stages, the granulosa cells divide and grow forming multiple layers. Granulosa cells have receptors for LH and follicle-stimulating hormone (FSH) and their main function is the production of estrogen. During the follicular phase the oocyte grows from 15 μm to 135 μm and becomes one of the biggest cells in the body. It matures and starts secreting glycoproteins forming the zona pellucida (pale zone). The considerable size is explained by the fact that the oocyte must possess all machinery (mitochondria, nutrients, etc) to sustain the pregnancy until implantation occurs. The cells outside the

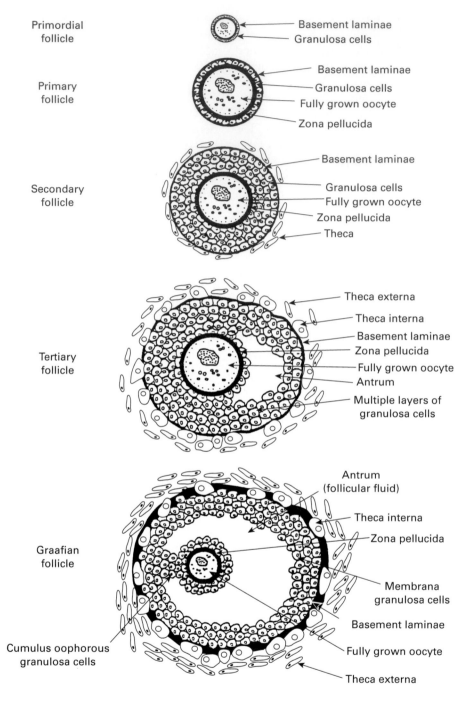

Figure 1.5 Structure of the ovarian follicle during growth and development. Reproduced from Erickson GF, Magoffin DA, Dyer CA, Hofeditz C. The ovarian androgen producing cells: a review of stucture/function relationships. *Endocr Rev* 1985;6:371–99, with permission of The Endocrine Society

Table 1.1 Some non-steroidal factors produced by the ovary

Non-steroidal factor	Proposed function
Activin	Stimulates FSH release
Follistatin	Suppresses FSH release
Inhibin	Inhibits FSH release
Angiogenic factors	Vascularization of corpus luteum
FRP	Follicle atresion, aromatase inhibin
Growth factors	Modulation of steroidogenesis
FSH binding inhibitor	Inhibits binding of FSH to receptor
LH binding inhibitor	Inhibits binding of LH to receptor
Müllerian inhibiting factor	Development of reproductive tract
Oxytocin (corpus luteum)	Modulates progesterone secretion and life span of corpus luteum
Relaxin	Remodeling of reproductive tract
Renin–angiotensin	Ovulation; regulation of steroidogenesis

FRP, follicular-regulating protein; FSH, follicle-stimulating hormone; LH, luteinizing hormone

follicle also grow and differentiate forming the thecal layers. The tertiary follicle has a fluid-filled space named the antrum (hence antral follicle). The fluid consists of plasma filtrate and secretory products of the granulosa cells.

Under the influence of FSH, the antral follicles grow further to form mature Graafian follicles. The antral fluid increases in volume and the oocyte is surrounded by a clump of granulosa cells called the cumulus oophorus. At this stage, the follicle is at least 14 mm in mean diameter and is ready to release the egg. The resumption of meiosis occurs following the preovulatory surge of LH.

The ovarian stroma consists of three cell types: contractile cells, connective tissue cells and interstitial cells. The interstitial cells secrete steroid hormones, mainly androgens, and undergo morphologic changes in response to LH and human chorionic gonadotropin (hCG). As the follicle develops, the interstitial cells differentiate and become thecal cells. After ovulation, blood vessels invade the cavity of the follicle. Granulosa cells and thecal cells transform into granulosa–lutein and theca–lutein cells and form the corpus luteum. The corpus luteum secretes estrogen and progesterone. In the absence of pregnancy, the corpus luteum undergoes degeneration to form the corpus albicans. The ovary also produces a number of other substances in addition to steroid hormones. Some of these are described in Table 1.1.

The pelvic floor and support of the pelvic organs

The pelvic organs and the abdominal content of a woman are supported via intricate systems of muscles and ligaments. There is still debate among anatomists, physiologists, urologists and urogynecologists with regard to the role that various structures play in the support of the pelvic organs. We are not going to join this debate but will merely list some structures which have been universally accepted as important. The pelvic opening is closed by the perineal body and muscles, the biggest and most important of which is the levator ani. This muscle originates from the side walls of the pelvis and is funnel shaped. The funnel has three orifices: urethra, vagina and anus. The uterus is held in place largely by the uterosacral and cardinal ligaments and to a lesser extend by the round and broad

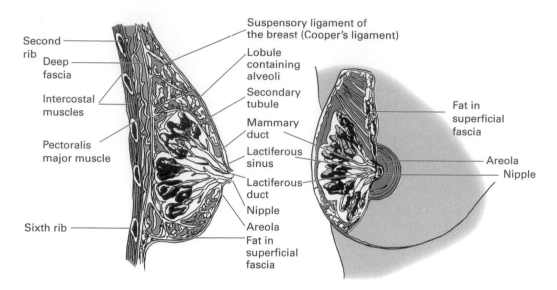

Figure 1.6 Cross-section of the breast. Reproduced with permission from Tortora GJ, Grabowski SR, Schmidt Prezbindowski K, eds. *Principles of Human Anatomy and Physiology*, 10th edn. New York: John Wiley & Sons, 2002:1040

Table 1.2 Hormonal regulation of the breast

Ductal growth
  Estrogen
  Cortisol
  Growth hormone
Alveolar growth
  Progesterone
  Prolactin
  Growth hormone
  Cortisol
Lactation
  Prolactin
  Placental lactogen
  Cortisol
  Insulin
  Insulin-like growth factor

ligaments. Prolapse of the pelvic organs depends on (1) how well developed the support systems are (e.g., as a result of genetic endowment and exercise) and (2) the stresses put onto them via increased intra-abdominal pressure, stretching the tearing (pregnancy, childbirth, obesity, constipation, ascites, chronic cough, etc).

The breast

The breast is situated between the second and the sixth rib horizontally (Figure 1.6) and between the parasternal area and the mid-axillary area vertically. The central thickness of the breast is between 5 and 7 cm. It has various configurations: in young nulliparous females it has a conical appearance, and in parous women and later in life it becomes pendulous. The nipple is situated near the summit of the breast, usually at the level of the fourth intercostal space. The breast extends upward and laterally toward the axilla, a part of which is known as the axillary tail of Spence. The average breast weighs about 100 g and often there is discrepancy in size with the left breast usually being bigger. In pregnancy, the breast increases dramatically in size and weighs three to four times more than in the non-pregnant state. The structure of the breast consists of skin, subcutaneous tissue and the stroma. The skin is thin, flexible and elastic, which allows the breast to expand and shrink depending on the physiologic condition. The breast skin has hair, sebaceous glands and eccrine sweat glands. Below the skin, there is connective tissue which includes the fatty tissue, blood vessels, nerves and lymphatics. Within the stroma, there is a ductal–lobular–alveolar structure which resembles a river and its tributaries. Proximally, the alveoli are very small, but distally they increase in size and open into the lactiferous sinuses, just below the areola structure. There are 15 to 25 lobes, each one consisting of multiple lobules, and each lobule has hundreds of tubulosaccular secretory units. The nipple is a conical elevation where 15 to 25 milk ducts open. It has a rich sensory nerve supply and sebaceous and apocrine sweat glands. The areola surrounds the nipple and can vary in size from 1.5 to 5 cm, and peripherally there are Morgagni's tubercles which are openings of the sebaceous glands of Montgomery. During stimulation, the nipple becomes erect and the areola constricts; both are caused by the underlying smooth muscle. The breast tissue is attached to the overlying skin via a subcutaneous fascia known as Cooper's suspensory ligaments. The bottom of the breast lies on the pectoralis fascia. The blood supply to the breasts is via the internal mammary artery (60% of the blood), lateral thoracic artery (25–30%) and the intercostal arteries (5–10%). The lymphatics of the breast are quite numerous and mainly go toward the axilla and along the internal mammary artery. There are, however, communications with the other breast, with subdiaphragmatic and intraperitoneal lymph nodes and with the liver.

The sensory nerve supply of the breast is derived from the fourth, fifth and sixth intercostal nerves. The same nerves carry sympathetic fibres with them to the breast.

The alveolar unit is the milk-producing structure of the breast and it has three types of cells: alveolar cells, chief cells and myoepithelial cells. The alveolar cells are stimulated by sex steroids and are responsible for milk production. The chief cells provide the energy source for the alveolar cells. The myoepithelial cells are of ectodermal origin, respond to oxytocin by constriction and allow the expression of milk. The stromal tissue is quiescent until puberty, when the breasts start developing in an orderly manner first described by Marshall and Tanner. Breast development usually starts between 9 and 11 years of age, together with pubic and axillary hair growth. It is difficult to outline precisely the relative contribution of the numerous hormonal and growth factor influences on breast growth (see Table 1.2). *In vitro* estrogen appears to stimulate the ductal proliferation, while progesterone stimulates lobulo-alveolar development. The breast undergoes cyclic changes associated with ovulation, and premenstrual breasts can be engorged and tender probably because of tissue edema and hyperemia.

Before pregnancy, the breast consists mainly of ducts, connective tissue and adipose tissue. During pregnancy, lobulo-alveolar elements differentiate under the influence of sex hormone but also placental lactogen, prolactin, insulin and insulin-like growth factor.

Hormones in reproduction

2

Nikolai Manassiev and Henry Burger

INTRODUCTION

A number of hormones and hormone-like substances are involved in regulating the reproductive process in humans. Some are well studied, others less so. It is not our aim to discuss all of them. In this chapter we will restrict our discussion to those hormones whose structure and function have been well studied and are universally accepted.

LUTEINIZING HORMONE-RELEASING HORMONE

The neurohormone involved in regulating the synthesis and release of both follicle-stimulating hormone (FSH) and luteinizing hormone (LH) is gonadotropin-releasing hormone (GnRH), also known as luteinizing hormone-releasing hormone (LHRH). It is a decapeptide secreted from the LHRH neurons of the hypothalamus into the portal vessels. LHRH modulates both LH and FSH, neither of them selectively. The half-life of LHRH is 2–4 min. It is secreted as a pulse every hour during the follicular phase and every 3 h during the luteal phase. Its main function is to promote synthesis, storage and release of gonadotropins. Pulsatile secretion of LHRH leads to pulsatile release of LH and FSH. Therefore, hypothalamic LHRH neurons regulate the synthesis and secretion of FSH and LH by the anterior pituitary. Alteration of the output of FSH and LH can be achieved by increasing or decreasing the amplitude or frequency of LHRH pulses.

FOLLICLE-STIMULATING HORMONE AND LUTEINIZING HORMONE

FSH and LH are responsible primarily for the processes concerned with follicular and germ cell development and with ovulation. LH and FSH are secreted by the gonadotrophic cells (basophilic), which comprise about 10% of the anterior pituitary. LH and FSH are hetero-dimeric glycoprotein hormones of similar size, and consist of a common α chain and a distinct β chain. The same α chain is present in thyroid-stimulating hormone (TSH) and human chorionic gonadotropin (hCG). The α subunit is encoded by a single gene located on chromosome 6, while the FSH β subunit is located on chromosome 11 and the LH β subunit on chromosome 19. FSH has a longer half-life than LH (Table 2.1). Secretion of LH and FSH is under the control of LHRH, which, as mentioned above, is secreted in a pulsatile fashion. LH is released in pulses at a frequency of every 60–90 min during the follicular phase and every 3 h during the luteal phase. The mechanism of FSH and LH action involves binding to specific cell membrane receptors and subsequent activation of the adenylate cyclase system, which in turn leads to signaling steps within the cell.

FSH receptors are present only on granulosa cells. FSH stimulates the growth and division of the granulosa cells of the ovarian follicle and controls the aromatase responsible for estradiol formation within these cells. It also induces the synthesis of LH receptors on the granulosa cells and is involved in the production of inhibin, activin and insulin-like growth factor I. LH stimulates the ovarian theca cells to produce androgens, which diffuse to the granulosa cells where they are converted into estrogens. Plasma estradiol peaks before the LH surge, which, in turn, triggers ovulation. Postovulation LH contributes to the formation of the corpus luteum. Once conception has occurred, pituitary gonadotropins are no longer required to sustain the pregnancy.

ESTRADIOL, PROGESTERONE AND FEEDBACK CONTROL OF FOLLICLE-STIMULATING HORMONE AND LUTEINIZING HORMONE SECRETION

The plasma concentrations of circulating FSH and LH increase markedly after the menopause or after surgical castration. This rise is attributable to the decline of estradiol and inhibin (mainly inhibin B) secretion. Administration of physiologic doses of estradiol mimicking those found in the follicular phase of the menstrual cycle in reproductive aged women leads to a decline of FSH and LH to levels approximately 50% of the postmenopausal level. This is an example of classic negative feedback in premenopausal women. It requires a relatively small rise from low circulating levels of estradiol for an effect on FSH and LH to be observed. Furthermore, the effect of estradiol is seen very quickly. However, because inhibin is not administered in hormone replacement therapy (HRT) the postmenopausal FSH and LH values do not return to within the premenopausal range with HRT. In regularly menstruating women, if plasma concentration of estradiol increases two- to four-fold and this increase is sustained over 48 h or so, then LH and FSH secretion is enhanced, not suppressed. This is termed positive feedback. The most important effect of progesterone is that high plasma levels of this hormone enhance the negative feedback of estradiol and suppress FSH and LH secretion to a very low level. By contrast, low levels may enhance the positive feedback of estradiol.

PROLACTIN

The hormone prolactin is produced by the lactotrophic cells (acidophilic) of the anterior pituitary. It constitutes 15–20% of the normal pituitary and this increases to 70% during pregnancy. Prolactin has a single polypeptide chain containing 198 amino acids. The gene for prolactin production is on chromosome 6. The hormone is essential for lactation and a mass of the receptors for this hormone is present in the human breast and gonads. It may also have some function in the regulation of steroidogenesis in the ovary. The plasma levels vary during the day, the highest plasma concentration occurring during sleep. Under normal circumstances, prolactin secretion is restrained by the hypothalamus and the inhibitory factor for prolactin appears to be dopamine. Prolactin release is stimulated by sleep, estrogen, suckling, stimulation of the nipple, thyrotropin-releasing hormone (TRH), stress, opiates and anti-dopamine medications. Some of the properties of LHRH, LH, FSH and prolactin are summarized in Table 2.1.

OVARIAN STEROIDS

Four major classes of steroids are derived from cholesterol: the progestogens, the androgens, the estrogens and the corticosteroids. The ovary is involved in the synthesis and secretion of the first three (Figure 2.1).

Natural progestogens are characterized by possessing 21 carbons (C-21 steroids), androgens by being comprised of 19 carbons (C-19 steroids), and natural estrogens have 18 carbons (C-18 steroids) in their structure. Ovarian steroids can exert feedback on both the hypothalamus and the pituitary. Whether estrogens and progestogens stimulate or inhibit gonadotropin release depends upon the plasma level and the duration of exposure. The plasma concentrations, production rates and secretion rates of the main ovarian steroids are given in Table 2.2.

Over 97–98% of the steroids secreted by the ovary are bound to plasma proteins. Testosterone is mainly bound to sex hormone-binding

Table 2.1 Properties of human luteinizing hormone, luteinizing hormone-releasing hormone, follicle-stimulating hormone and prolactin[*]

Hormone	Secreted from	Acts upon	Composition	Distribution half-life[†] in blood (min)	Levels in human blood (U/l)
LHRH	Hypothalamus (preoptic area and arcuate nucleus)	Anterior pituitary	Decapeptide	2–4	N/A
LH	Anterior pituitary gonadotrophs (basophilic)	Thecal cells; granulosa cells; luteal cells; interstitial cells	Glycoprotein, α chain 89 aminoacids; β chain 115 amino acids, 1 carbohydrate chain	30–60[**]	Male > 12 years 5–12 U/l Female Early follicular 0.4–15 IU/l Midcycle 20–70 IU/l Luteal 0.4–15 IU/l Menopause 20–70 IU/l
FSH	As LH	Granulosa cells	Glycoprotein, α chain identical to LH; β chain 115 amino acids, 2 carbohydrate chains	120–150[**]	Male (age 13–70) 1.2–16 IU/l Female Early follicular 2–8 IU/l Midcycle 2.7–27 IU/l Luteal 1.2–7.3 IU/l Menopause 18–93 IU/l
Prolactin	Anterior pituitary lactotrophs (acidophilic)	Ovarian follicles; luteal cells; mammary glands	Polypeptide single chain of 198 amino acids	10–20	Male and female 60–450 U/l

LHRH, luteinizing hormone-releasing hormone; N/A, not available; LH, luteinizing hormone;
FSH, follicle-stimulating hormone
[*]Values vary from one laboratory to another
[**]Elimination half-life: LH, 10–12 h; FSH, 17 ± 3h
[†]Distribution half-life and biological half-life are different concepts. For the reproductive hormones the biological half-life is greater than the distribution half-life

globulin (SHBG). Estradiol is bound to albumin (60%) and SHBG (38%). SHBG is a β-globulin formed in the liver with a molecular weight of about 95 000. The level of SHBG, and thus the level of free hormone, can be affected by a number of conditions. Levels are increased by estradiol, combined oral contraceptives (COCs) and thyroid hormones, and are decreased by androgens, hypothyroidism and obesity.

There are number of naturally occurring gonadal steroids, all of them with different potency. The ones that are most important for clinical practice and their principal actions on the reproductive system are outlined in Table 2.3. In our discussion we are going to use the terms progesterone and estrogen or estradiol to denote all naturally occurring progestogens and estrogens.

Mechanism of action of steroid hormones

All ovarian steroids have the same basic mechanism of action. For clarity and because the estrogen activity has been widely studied,

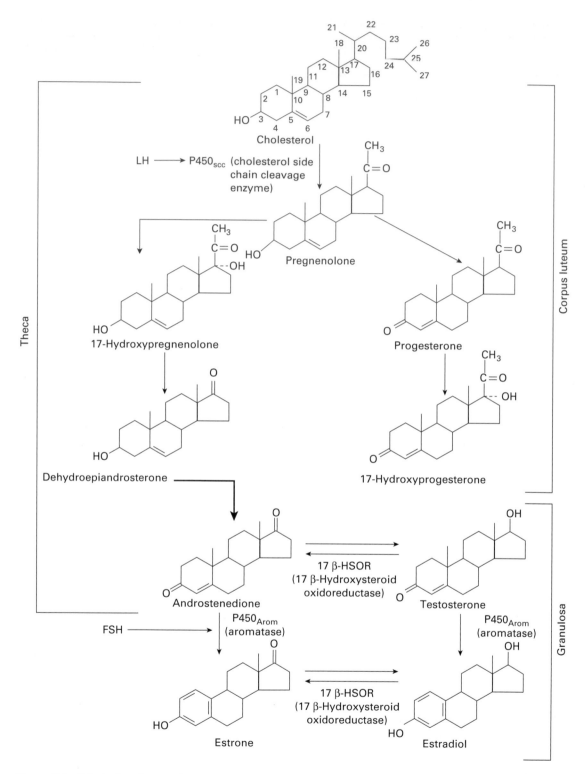

Figure 2.1 Principal pathways of steroid hormone biosynthesis in the human ovary. Reproduced from Carr BR. Disorders of the ovary and female reproductive tract. In Wilson JD, Foster DW, eds. *William's Textbook of Endocrinology*, 8th edn. Philadelphia, PA: W.B. Saunders, 1992:733–98, Copyright (1992), with permission from Elsevier

Table 2.2 Concentration, production rates and ovarian secretion rates of steroids in blood

Compound	Menstrual cycle phase	Representative concentration in plasma (nmol/l)	PR* (mg/day)	SR** by both ovaries (mg/day)
Estradiol	Early follicular	0.2 (200 pmol/l)	0.08	0.07
	Late follicular	1.2–2.6	0.5–1.0	0.4–0.8
	Midluteal	0.7 (700 pmol/l)	0.270	0.250
	Menopause	< 0.11 (110 pmol/l)		
Progesterone	Follicular	3.0	2.1	1.5
	Luteal	30–100	25	24
Testosterone		1.3 (0.5–2.8)	0.25–0.5	0.2–0.5
Androstenedione		5.6	3.2	0.8–1.6
Dehydroepiandrosterone		17	8.0	0.3–3

*PR, production rate, consisting of the sum of secretion rate and amount contributed by interconversion of precursor steroids; †SR, secretion rate, being the secretion of ovarian steroids in units per day

Table 2.3 Relative potency and principal actions of some naturally occurring sex steroids in females

Type of steroid and relative potency*	Properties
Estrogens	
17β-Estradiol (100%)	Stimulate secondary sexual characteristics
Estrone (10%)	Prepare the genital tract for spermatozoal transport
Estriol (1%)	Stimulate growth and the activity of mammary glands
	Stimulate the growth of the endometrium and prepare the endometrium for progesterone action
	Associated with sexual behavior
	Regulate secretion of gonadotropins
Progestogens	
Progesterone (100%)	Prepare uterus to receive embryo
17α-Hydroxyprogesterone (40–70%)	Maintain uterus during early pregnancy
	Stimulate growth of mammary glands but suppress the secretion of milk
	Regulate secretion of gonadotropins
Androgens	
5α-Dihydrotestosterone (100%)	Induce growth of androgen-dependent body hair
Testosterone (50%)	Influence sexual and aggressive behavior
Dehydroepiandrosterone (4%)	? Regulate secretion of gonadotropins

*The relative potencies are approximations only. They vary with (1) the assay used; (2) the affinity of the steroid for the steroid receptor in different tissues; (3) the local enzymatic conversion of the steroids in the target tissues; and (4) the differences in systemic metabolism

the mode of action described here uses estrogen as the example (Figure 2.2). Free steroids are thought to diffuse passively to all cells because there is no evidence as yet of an active transport mechanism. Steroids are preferentially retained in target cells as stable complexes bound to intracellular receptor proteins (i.e., estrogen receptor – ER), which are steroid- and tissue specific. The receptor is thought to be a hormone- or ligand-activated transcription factor. The terms are used interchangeably.

17

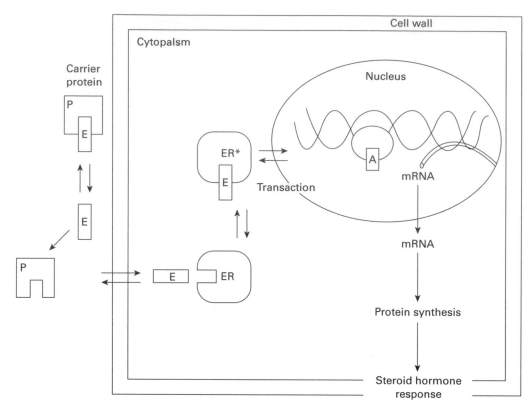

Figure 2.2 A schematic representation of the subcellular effects of estrogen (E) in estrogen target tissue. Estrogens dissociate from plasma proteins (P), bind to the estrogen receptor (ER) and the complex becomes activated (ER*). Activated ER complex interacts with the nuclear acceptor site on the DNA (A). This results in the activation of DNA polymerase and RNA polymerase to initiate subsequent cell proliferation and protein synthesis, respectively. The receptor is then destroyed (processed), in which case a new cytoplasmic receptor is synthesized or recycled for subsequent ligand binding. Whether the binding of estrogen and the receptor occurs on the cytoplasm in the nucleus has been debated. It is currently thought that the interaction happens in the nucleus. Reproduced from Manassiev N, Keating F, Whitehead M. Selective estrogen receptor modulators: a review for the clinician. In Studd J, ed. *The Management of the Menopause. The Millennium Review 2000*. Carnforth, UK: Parthenon Publishing, 2000:69–84

The ER has six structural domains (protein regions having some distinct feature or role), A to F, but the important ones are the steroid-binding domain and the DNA-binding domain. The receptor binds the hormone, i.e., estrogen, through its steroid-binding domain. The binding of the steroid by the receptor results in the activation of the receptor molecules, which leads to conformational changes in the hormone–receptor complex, including its DNA-binding domain. This activation allows the hormone–receptor complex to bind to specific sites in the DNA, termed nuclear acceptor sites. Once bound to the DNA, the activated steroid–receptor complex acts as a transcription factor, which 'switches on' genes, coding for the production of new proteins. The newly synthesized proteins change the metabolism of the target cell in a steroid-specific manner. The transfer of the steroid in the cell and nuclear binding of the steroid–receptor complex is rapid, occurring within minutes. Nuclear binding affects messenger RNA levels and synthesis within several hours, and finally protein synthesis and turnover happens within 12–24 h. The major physiologic effects of steroids in cells are seen in 12–36 h.

There are two estrogen receptors so far described: ERα (classic ER) and ERβ (recently described). Classic ER was cloned and sequenced from human breast cancer cells in

1986. The ERα consists of 595 aminoacids with a molecular weight of 66 kDa. The ERβ was cloned in 1996 from rat prostate and ovary. It consists of 485 amino acids and has a molecular weight of 54.2 kDa. ERβ is 95% homologous with ERα in the DNA-binding domain and 55% in the hormone-binding domain. ERα resides no chromosome 6 and ERβ on chromosome 14. ERα has a higher affinity for short-acting estrogens such as 17α-estradiol. Tissue distribution of ERα and ERβ varies and is under intense scientific investigation. Most of the work has been done on rodents, so-called estrogen receptor knockout (ERKO) mice. A knockout mouse is a genetically engineered animal in which the genome has been altered by site-directed recombination so that a particular gene is deleted. The reported findings may not be directly applicable to humans. The results depend on the sensitivity of the assays and are sometimes conflicting. Recent reports describe ERα predominance in the vagina, uterus, ovarian stroma, breast, cardiovascular system, liver, skeletal muscle, pituitary and epididymis; in contrast, ERβ is predominantly found in ovarian granulosa cells and the prostate. Both receptors are well represented in the brain and bone, but in different structural and functional parts. The levels of ERα and ERβ may vary depending on the age of the animal. The physiologic role of the different receptors is currently being studied. For example, ERα knockout mice develop to maturity, but are infertile, do not exhibit female sexual behavior and do not respond to estradiol.

Physiologic functions of steroid hormones

The main function of the ovarian steroids is related to reproduction. They are instrumental in developing the secondary sexual characteristics, establishing the menstrual cycle and in maintaining pregnancy. However, as our methods for studying the steroid hormones have developed, so has our understanding of their wider functions.

Estrogen

Female maturation Estrogen stimulates the growth of the vagina, uterus and fallopian tubes and the secondary sexual characteristics during puberty. It stimulates fat deposition, stromal development and ductal growth of the breast and is responsible for the accelerated growth phase and the closing of the epiphyses of the long bones that occurs at puberty. Estrogen contributes to the growth of axillary and pubic hair and alters the distribution of the body fat so as to produce the typical female body habitus. It stimulates the pigmentation of the skin, most prominent in the region of the nipples and areolae and in the genital region.

Other biological effects of estrogen Estrogen exerts effects on the cardiovascular system, connective tissue and numerous aspects of the metabolism such as lipids and carbohydrate metabolism. Some of those effects are well established and important and some are less well studied and/or less significant. Some estrogenic effects are summarized in Table 2.4.

The main sources of estrogen in women are the granulosa cells and the luteinied granulosa and theca cells of the ovaries. Estrogen is also produced by fat tissue and, in smaller amounts, by muscle and nervous tissue. Estrone and estriol are mostly formed from estradiol in the liver.

Progesterone

The chief function of progesterone is to prepare the endometrium for acceptance and maintenance of pregnancy, and the stimulation of alveolar growth of the mammary glands. Some of the effects of progesterone are listed in Table 2.5. Progesterone is produced by theca and granulosa lutein cells and the corpus luteum.

Androgens

Androgen production in the female is greater than is widely appreciated. The role of androgens in the female includes acting as precursors

19

Table 2.4 Biological effects of estrogen

Reproductive system
Gonadotropin regulation
Stimulation of secondary sexual characteristics
Increasing cervical mucus production
Breast development (stromal and ductal tissue)
Modulation of sexual behavior
Endometrial stimulation

Cardiovascular system
Increased cardiac output
Vasodilatation
Endothelial effects
Suppression of appetite
Stimulates skin growth and wound healing
Reduces motility of the bowel
Mild anabolic effect

Metabolic effects
Higher levels of corticosteroid-binding globulin,
  thyroxin-binding globulin, SHBG, renin
Reduction of cholesterol
Reduction of bone resorption
Reduction of capillary fragility
Promotion of coagulation

SHBG, sex hormone-binding globulin

Table 2.5 Biological effects of progesterone

Reproductive system
  gonadotropin regulation
  endometrial decidualization
  maintenance of early pregnancy
  breast development (alveolar tissue)
Increase of appetite
Mild catabolic effect
Increase of basal body temperature via
  thermoregulatory centre of the hypothalamus
Binding to the aldosterone receptor in the kidney and
  promoting natriuresis
Contributes to premenstrual symptoms such as
  bloatedness, heavy tender breasts
Slows peristalsis in the gastrointestinal tract, which may
  cause constipation
Depressant and hypnotic effects on the brain
Alters the function of the respiratory centre (increases
  respiratory drive)

Table 2.6 Biological effects of androgens

Reproductive system
  libido, sexual behavior
  growth of androgen-dependent body hair
  ? regulation of gonadotropins
Anabolic effect
  nitrogen retention
  muscle growth
Stimulate bone formation
Increase serum production
Increase EPO production
Decrease HDL cholesterol
Contribute to general well-being

EPO, erythropoietin; HDL, high-density lipoprotein

for estrogen production, anabolic effects, stimulation of axillary and pubic hair growth, sebum production, stimulation of bone formation, and stimulation of production of erythropoietin (EPO) from the kidneys (Table 2.6).

Androgens are produced from the ovaries, the adrenal glands and from peripheral conversion in adipose tissue. During reproductive life, the relative contribution from these sources varies. The ovaries and adrenals produce androstenedione, testosterone and dehydroepiandrosterone (DHEA), and the adrenals also produce DHEA sulfate (DHEAS). Androstenedione, DHEA and DHEAS are converted peripherally to testosterone, dihydrotestosterone (DHT) and estrogen. Only 1–2% of the total circulating testosterone is free or biologically active, the rest being bound to SHBG and albumin. In women, there are alterations in the level because SHBG has a dramatic effect on the free levels in plasma, binding 66% of total circulating testosterone. SHBG is increased by increased levels of estradiol and thyroxine, and suppressed by testosterone, glucocorticoids, excessive growth hormone, high insulin levels and obesity. The daily androstenedione and testosterone production in premenopausal women is thought to be about 3.2 mg and 0.26 mg, respectively.

In premenopausal women, 25% of testosterone is produced by the ovaries, 25% by the adrenals and 50% by peripheral conversion. In postmenopausal women, 50% of testosterone is produced by the ovaries, 10% by the adrenals and 40% by peripheral conversion, and the overall androgen production decreases with age. The age-related decrease in androgen production starts premenopausally and testosterone levels fall by approximately 50% between the ages of 20 and 40, and then level off. After the menopause, the process continues and the age-related decline is particularly noticeable for DHEA and DHEAS. Following natural menopause, the level of androstenedione is 50% of the premenopausal value. After oophorectomy, the levels of testosterone and androstenedione fall by 50% in previously premenopausal women and by 50% and 21% respectively in previously post-menopausal women. Some androgenic effects are listed in Table 2.6.

INHIBINS, ACTIVINS AND FOLLISTATINS

Inhibins, activins and follistatins are produced by the ovary and are a part of a larger family of growth factors. Inhibins are proteins that consist of a common α subunit and one of two β subunits (β_A or β_B). They are classified as inhibin A if they contain β_A chain or inhibin B if they contain β_B chain. Activins are proteins that have two β chains (homodimers β_A/β_A, β_B/β_B; or heterodimers – β_A/β_B) but no α chains.

Inhibin A is mainly produced by the dominant follicle and the subsequent corpus luteum. It is maintained at relatively constant low levels through most of the follicular phase, then exhibits a late follicular phase rise (in keeping with its production by the dominant follicle), a midcycle peak, and a long peak with the highest levels recorded during the luteal phase. Inhibin A appears to exert negative feedback on FSH during the luteal phase of the cycle.

Inhibin B is found in the granulosa cells of antral follicles during the end of the luteal phase of the preceding cycle and the early follicular phase of the next; its concentration in plasma changes in parallel with FSH: it rises in the early follicular phase, declines toward midcycle, shows a midcycle peak and reaches its lowest level during the luteal phase. This suggests it is produced by the cohort of small antral follicles and suppresses FSH in the follicular phase. Inhibin B is currently being evaluated as a test for ovarian reserve (the ability of the ovary to produce oocyte(s) in response to stimulation with fertility drugs).

Inhibin A, together with α-fetoprotein and free β-hCG, shows much promise in serologic testing for Down's syndrome in early pregnancy. Activins and follistatins are less well studied. As the names suggest, one property of the activins is to enhance the secretion of FSH, while follistatins suppress it by binding and inactivating the activins. Their role as gonadal feedback regulators is still under investigation.

The female reproductive cycle   3

Nikolai Manassiev and Henry Burger

INTRODUCTION

From the reproductive point of view the female lifecycle can be conveniently divided into three parts: from birth to menarche, from menarche to menopause, and the post-menopause era. Definitions of various terms used in reproductive medicine are given in Table 3.1. A graphical representation of some of these definitions is shown in Figure 3.1.

HORMONE SECRETION: FROM INFANCY THROUGH PUBERTY

In the female, luteinizing hormone (LH) and follicle-stimulating hormone (FSH) levels are elevated at birth but fall to low levels within a few months and remain low throughout the prepubertal years, with FSH generally slightly higher than LH. Steroid hormones, such as dehydroepiandrosterone (DHEA), estradiol and testosterone, are increased at birth; then they decrease to very low levels.

The adrenal androgens DHEA and DHEA sulfate (DHEAS) begin to increase several years before puberty. This increase may be important in initiating pubic and axillary hair growth (adrenarche) and other pubertal events.

Puberty

The sequence of events by which a child reaches sexual maturity with the development of secondary sexual characteristics and an associated growth spurt is called puberty. The mechanisms initiating puberty are unclear. There has been a secular trend toward an earlier menarche in girls in Western Europe and the USA. It is generally agreed that during the last 100 years or so, the age at which girls first menstruate has decreased to between 12

Table 3.1 Definitions of various terms used in reproductive medicine

Puberty: the sequence of events by which a child reaches sexual maturity with development of secondary sexual characteristics and an associated growth spurt

Menarche: first menses (mean age 13 years, range 10.5–16)

Precocious puberty: the onset of sexual maturation before age 8

Delayed puberty:
  no breast development by age 13
  no pubic hair by age 14
  more than 5 years between breast development and menarche
  no menstruation by age 16

Reproductive life: the period from menarche to menopause

Menopause: permanent cessation of menses (at least 12 months after last menstrual period). In the UK the mean age at menopause is 51 years (range 45–55)

Premature menopause: menopause at or before age 40

Early menopause: menopause after age 40, but before age 45

Late menopause: menopause at or after age 55

Perimenopause: period of declining ovarian function (mean age at beginning of clinical symptoms 47 years). It begins with stage – 2 and ends 12 months after the final menstrual period. It is often used interchangeably with menopause transition

Climacteric: the period from decreasing to absent ovarian function (used synonymously with perimenopause). It is desirable to use the terms perimenopause and climacteric only in discussion with patients and not in scientific publications

Menopausal transition: stages – 2 and – 1. It ends with the final menstrual period, i.e., it can be recognized only after 12 months of amenorrhea

Postmenopause: the years after the final menstrual period (stages + 1 and + 2). However, the terms 'postmenopause' and 'menopause' are often used interchangeably

and 13 years. In Western Europe, the age of menarche decreased by four months for each decade between 1850 and 1950 but has not

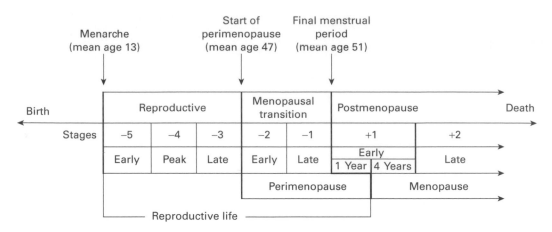

Figure 3.1 Graphical representation of various terms used in reproductive medicine. Data derived from Soules MR, Sherman S, Parrott E, *et al*. Executive Summary: Stages of Reproductive Aging Workshop (STRAW). *Fertil Steril* 2001; 76:874–8

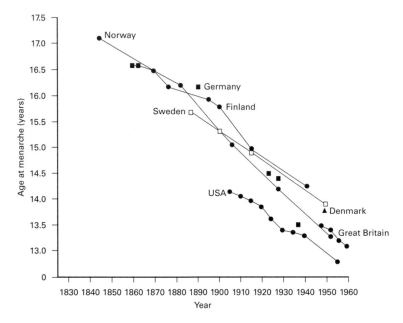

Figure 3.2 Secular trend towards an earlier age at menarche in girls from Western Europe and the USA. Reproduced with permission from Johnson MH, Everitt BJ. *Essential Reproduction*, 2nd edn. Oxford: Blackwell Scientific Publishers, 1984:157

decreased during the last four decades (Figure 3.2). The mean age at menarche for girls in the United States is 12.8 years. It can occur as early as 10 and as late as 16 years. Menarche is preceded by breast budding, sexual hair growth and a growth spurt. For several years after menarche the menstrual cycles may be anovulatory and variable in frequency, duration and heaviness of menstrual flow.

There are a number of factors that might have contributed to the earlier attainment of sexual maturity and that give an insight into the mechanisms controlling the initiation of puberty.

Table 3.2 Stages of follicular development

Follicular phase: variable length, average 11–17 days

(1) Recruitment: days 1–4
(2) Selection: days 5–7
(3) Dominance: days 8–12; ends with ovulation

Ovulation: hours

Luteal phase: relatively constant length, 13–15 days

Environment

Health care and personal health have improved over the years, along with living conditions and economic standards. These have certainly contributed to increased longevity, but their relationship to puberty is less clear. In Western societies, people are exposed to more light now than in the 19th century, thanks to the advent of electricity. Increased light exposure in some species can accelerate puberty, presumably through modulation within the central nervous system, mediated perhaps through the pineal gland and melatonin. Interestingly, contrary to expectation, blind girls experience an earlier menarche. Puberty occurs early among girls living in urban areas and in those whose mothers matured early.

Nutrition and body weight

Moderate obesity is associated with earlier menarche and menarche is commonly delayed in severely underweight and malnourished girls. Such observations suggest that critical body weight, or more specifically critical body fat, is necessary for menarche. In fact, the body weight at menarche over the past 100 years has remained surprisingly constant, at about 47 kg. The link between the critical body fat and puberty may be the hormone leptin, produced by the adipocytes. It has been suggested that a critical body leptin level is needed to kick-start the luteinizing hormone-releasing hormone (LHRH) neurons into activity.

The normal menstrual cycle during the reproductive years

The menstrual cycle during the reproductive years (from puberty to the menopause) is a complex event which depends on a timely and intricate interaction between the hypothalamus, the pituitary, the ovaries and the uterus. Its final common pathway is pregnancy or menstruation in the absence of pregnancy. There are numerous direct and indirect, positive and negative, autocrine and paracrine links between the main players. This makes the task of describing the menstrual cycle difficult. For practical purposes, it is easiest to concentrate mainly on the changes in the ovaries and the endometrium.

Ovarian cycle

The follicle is the engine of the ovarian cycle (Figure 3.3). Follicular development goes through several stages (Table 3.2; see also Figure 1.5) and each of these will be discussed in turn. Serum hormone changes during the menstrual cycle are summarized graphically in Figure 3.4.

Follicular phase The menstrual cycle begins with the first day of menstruation but follicular growth is initiated during the last few days of the luteal phase of the preceding menstrual cycle. Near the end of the previous luteal phase, plasma progesterone, estrogen and inhibin A levels decline because of the demise of the corpus luteum, and a rise of FSH occurs (days 1–4). FSH initiates the recruitment of a follicular cohort (of antral follicles). These follicles start developing and secreting steroid hormones as well as acquiring FSH and LH receptors. From the middle of the follicular phase onward, estrogen levels rise steadily, leading to an estradiol surge. In parallel with this increase, there is an increase in the levels of 17-α-hydroxyprogesterone, testosterone, androstenedione and inhibin. FSH levels begin to decline because of the negative

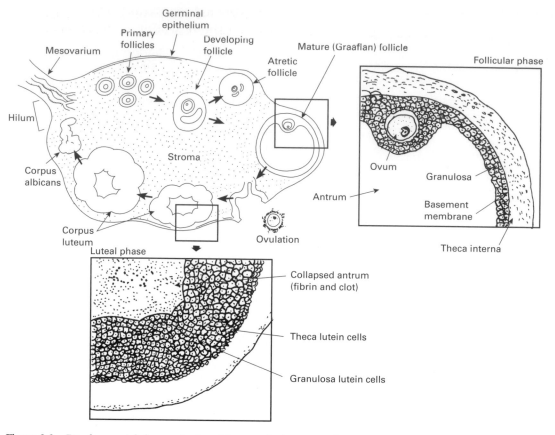

Figure 3.3 Developmental changes in the adult ovary during a complete menstrual cycle. Reproduced from Carr BR, Wilson JD. Disorders of the ovary and female reproductive tract. In Wilson JD, Braunwald E, Isselbacher KJ, *et al*., eds. *Harrison's Principles of Internal Medicine*, 12th edn. New York, NY: McGraw-Hill, 1991:1776–95

feedback of estrogens and particularly inhibin B secreted by the developing follicle. In response to the decline of the FSH, the development of adjacent follicles is inhibited (days 5–7). This leads to the preovulatory phase (days 8–12) during which FSH starts rising again. At the end of that phase LH surges, triggering ovulation. After the surge, LH, FSH and estradiol levels fall precipitously and progesterone and inhibin A levels start to rise. The first half of the cycle is complete. The length of the follicular phase varies and depends on the rate of maturation of the principal preantral follicle(s).

Ovulation Prior to ovulation, estrogen secretion by the preovulatory follicle increases dramatically and initiates the LH surge. The

prerequisite for the surge is an estradiol level of > 650 pmol/l or a doubling of the previous estradiol level for 48–50 h. LH initiates the process of luteinization of the granulosa cells and progesterone secretion. During the 34–36 h after the onset of the LH surge, ovulation occurs. The peak of the LH surge is 10–16 h prior to ovulation. The LH surge also initiates the resumption of meiosis in the oocyte, followed by the release of the first polar body. Prior to ovulation, a small protrusion of the follicular wall, called the stigma, appears and represents the location where a rupture occurs with the release of the oocyte–cumulus complex. The exact mechanism of the rupture of the follicle is unknown but it is believed to involve proteolytic enzymes, such as collagenase, plasmin and prostaglandins. In some cycles, the ovum is not released, which has

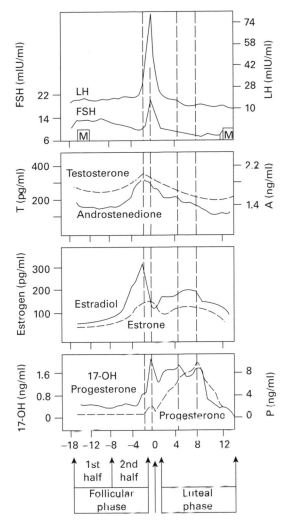

function. The granulosa cells change: they enlarge and become granulosa–lutein cells, surrounded by newly formed theca–lutein cells. They contain a yellow pigment (lipofuscin), hence the name lutein. The luteal phase of the cycle is characterized by rising plasma progesterone and 17-α-hydroxyprogesterone concentrations which peak around eight days after the LH surge, rising luteal estradiol and estrone levels which peak for a second time, to somewhat lesser levels, and then the pre-ovulatory peak. In the luteal phase, inhibin A level changes are parallel to the rise and fall of progesterone and estradiol. FSH, LH, testosterone and androstenedione levels decline to their lowest in the cycle. The nadir of FSH and LH is due to the negative feedback of estradiol, progesterone and inhibin A, and stops a new cohort of follicles from developing. Although the level of estradiol is relatively high, it does not produce a surge of LH and FSH because of the high levels of progesterone. If pregnancy does not occur, the corpus luteum function begins to decline rapidly nine to 11 days following ovulation, a process known as luteolysis. It leads to the formation of the fibrous scar, the corpus albicans. The levels of estradiol, progesterone and inhibin A fall, FSH starts to increase and a new cohort of follicles is recruited.

The functions of the corpus luteum are (1) to secrete progesterone, (2) to prepare the estrogen-primed endometrium for receiving a fertilized ovum, and (3) to maintain an early pregnancy. The corpus luteum is mainly under the influence of LH. However, LH or human chorionic gonadotropin (hCG) administration during the luteal phase of normal women can extend the functional life of the corpus luteum and the secretion of progesterone for up to two additional weeks. The length of the luteal phase is relatively constant at around 13–15 days.

Two-cell two-gonadotropin theory LH stimulates theca cells to produce C-19 steroids (mainly androstenedione and testosterone) from cholesterol. The steroids diffuse to the nearby granulosa cells (granulosa cells do not

Figure 3.4 Serum hormone levels during the human menstrual cycle. Adapted with permission from Johnson MH, Everitt BJ. *Essential Reproduction*, 2nd edn. Oxford: Blackwell Scientific Publishers, 1984:114

given rise to the concept of the luteinized unruptured follicle syndrome (LUFS), but the process appears to occur equally often in fertile, as well as infertile, women. However, women treated with high doses of prostaglandin synthetase inhibitors such as indomethacin may develop luteinized unruptured follicles. Women seeking fertility are advised to avoid the use of drugs that inhibit prostaglandin synthesis at the midcycle just prior to ovulation.

Luteal phase Following ovulation, the follicle undergoes marked changes in structure and

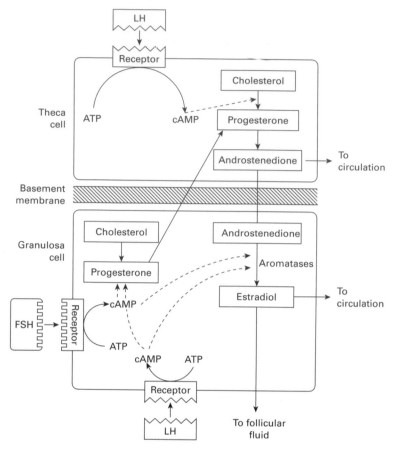

Figure 3.5 Two-cell, two-gonadotropin hypothesis of gonadotropin control of ovarian steroid biosynthesis. LH, luteinizing hormone; FSH, follicle-stimulating hormone. Adapted from Hsueh AJW, Adashi EY, Jones PBC, Welsh TH Jr. Hormonal regulation of the differentiation of culture ovarian granulosa cells. *Endocrine Rev* 1984;5:76, with permission of The Endocrine Society

possess a blood supply). FSH stimulates granulosa cells to aromatize the preformed androgens to produce estrogen (Figures 3.5 and 3.6). During the follicular stage, estrogen levels rise and parallel the growth of the follicle and the number of granulosa cells. After LH receptors have developed, the pre-ovulatory granulosa cells begin to secrete limited quantities of progesterone and 17-α-hydroxyprogesterone. Estradiol and progesterone exert positive feedback on the pituitary to augment LH release. Granulosa and theca cells change after ovulation to become the cells of the corpus luteum. They vascularize and start producing progesterone under the LH influence and continue the production of estradiol under the influence of FSH.

Non-steroidal hormones and growth factors are produced by the ovary and modulate steroid production. The concentration of ovarian steroids in follicular fluids exceeds concentration in blood many times.

Endometrial cycle

The hormonal changes during the cycle produce striking effects on the tissues of the reproductive tract. The most characteristic alterations occur in the endometrium. In the early proliferative phase, the endometrium is about 5 mm thick. The glands are narrow and tubular. The endometrium grows under the hormonal influence; in midcycle the thickness is 8–12 mm. Two days after ovulation, glycogen

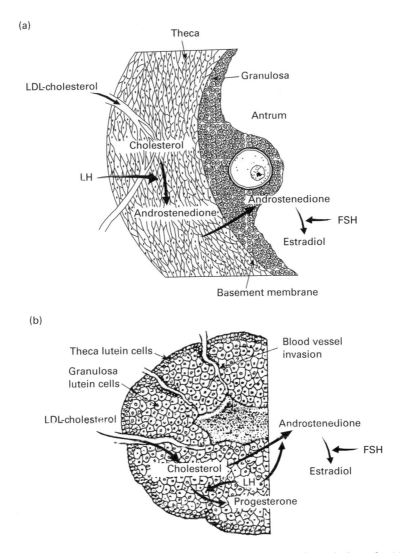

Figure 3.6 Cellular interactions in the ovary during the follicular phase (a) and luteal phase (b). LDL, low-density lipoprotein; FSH, follicle-stimulating hormone; LH, luteinizing hormone. Adapted from Carr BR, MacDonald PC, Simpson ER. The role of lipoproteins in the regulation of progesterone secretion by the human corpus luteum. *Fertil Steril* 1982;38:303–11, Copyright (1982), with permission from American Society for Reproductive Medicine

accumulates in the glands and they start to become tortuous and dilated. Intraluminal secretions are present, the endometrial stroma becomes edematous and the surrounding spiral arterioles enlarge. By day 27, the upper half of the endometrium is a solid sheet of well-developed decidual cells. In the absence of pregnancy, corpus luteum function ceases, with a resultant drop in estrogen and progesterone. There is now evidence that enzymes called matrix metalloproteinases play a role in endometrial shedding which gives rise to menstruation. Matrix metalloproteinases have the ability to degrade both interstitial matrix and basement membranes and are activated by estrogen and progesterone withdrawal. This results in necrosis of the endometrial blood vessels, prostaglandin release, endometrial ischemia and cell death. The endometrium breaks down and menstruation occurs. Menstrual flow consists of blood, desquamated endometrial tissues and exudate. The cervix

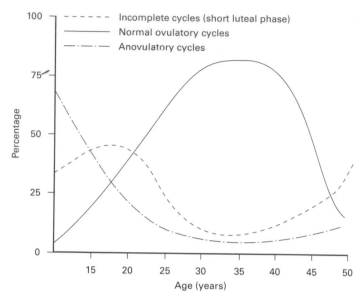

Figure 3.7 Relative incidence of three types of menstrual cycle with age of woman. Reproduced with permission from Johnson MH, Everitt BJ. *Essential Reproduction*, 2nd edn. Oxford: Blackwell Scientific Publishers, 1984:350

also undergoes cyclical changes. Those are described in more detail in Chapter 1.

Clinical menstrual cycle

Menstruation is the cyclic uterine bleeding experienced by most women of reproductive age. It represents the cyclic shedding of the secretory endometrium because of a decline in estradiol and progesterone production caused by a regressing corpus luteum.

The cycle length usually varies between one and two days each month, and only 50% of women have a cycle within the 26–30-day range that includes the so-called typical 28-day interval. The cycle length varies with age and ovulation (Figure 3.7). Anovulatory cycles tend to be shorter and occur during reproductive age.

The length of the normal menstrual cycle varies according to different authorities. One estimate is a mean of 26–28 days with a range of 21–35 days for ages between 17 and 41 years. The duration of menstruation is between 3 and 7 days with a total blood loss of up to 70–80 ml. When the menstrual blood loss exceeds 80 ml, there is good correlation with anemia (Hb < 12 g/l) and low plasma iron values. Since trying to determine the extent of menstrual blood loss relying on a patient's history is inaccurate, one practical way of estimating the menstrual loss is checking for anemia.

For most women, menstruation starts at the age of 13 years (normal range 10–16 years) and stops by 51 years (normal range 45–55 years).

The menopause and normal transition to menopause

The cessation of menstruation due to loss of ovarian function is called the menopause. In most women the menopause is not a sudden event but is preceded by a period of menstrual cycles of variable length called the perimenopause. The perimenopause begins with the first symptoms of the approaching menopause, i.e., vasomotor symptoms and menstrual irregularities, and ends 12 months after the last period. The perimenopause starts on average about four years before the last menstruation, with a mean age of 47 years. The terms perimenopause and menopause transition are often used interchangeably.

The aging of the ovary begins even before birth. Girls are born with a finite number of eggs. The number peaks at about 20 gestational weeks when there may be about 7 000 000 oogonia. The process of atresia then begins and the number is about 700 000 at birth and 250 000 to 400 000 at puberty. Atresia continues inexorably throughout adult life, which leads to an increasingly smaller and increasingly less responsive follicular pool. Postmenopausal ovaries contain atretic follicles only. The menopause occurs when the remaining ovarian follicles stop responding to FSH stimulation and the hormonal production of estrogen by therapy ceases.

Hormonal changes during the transition to menopause

The rate of follicular decline is linear until the age of approximately 36–38 years. Thereafter, the rate of depletion appears to accelerate. FSH shows a progressive increase from the age of 29–30 years onward, reflecting the diminishing number of follicles. Inhibin B decreases as the follicular pool is reduced. Low inhibin levels alter the negative feedback, thus allowing FSH to rise to stimulate the development of increasingly resistant follicles and to maintain estradiol levels. The remaining follicles mature irregularly, anovulatory cycles occur frequently and estrogen secretion becomes variable estrogen; but overall, the level of estrogen declines. Following the menopause, estradiol levels are commonly below 110 pmol/l and biochemically the menopause is said to occur with the elevation of FSH above 20–30 IU/l. In the postmenopause, estradiol levels decrease by 90% and estrone levels by 66%, leading to a reversal of the estradiol:estrone ratio to 1:3. The peripheral conversion of androstenedione to estrone increases and estrone becomes the primary estrogen of the postmenopause. The potency of this estrogen is less than 10% compared with that of estradiol. Consequently the classic symptoms of estrogen deficiency develop, as discussed below. Changes in androgens are more complex. Testosterone levels change little across the menopausal transition, androstenedione levels fall moderately and DHEA and DHEAS continue their age-related fall without any specific relationship to the menopause transition itself. By the age of 50–55 the levels of DHEA and DHEAS are 40% and 30% lower than young adult values, respectively, and those of androstenedione and testosterone 50% and 70% lower than young adult values, respectively. The net result of these changes is a relatively smaller decline in androgen as compared to estrogen. This has the following two effects: (1) a decrease in sex hormone-binding globulin (SHBG) and relatively higher levels of circulating androgens, and (2) the continuous exposure of the hair follicles to androgens. As a consequence, noticeable whiskers or sideburns may appear in postmenopausal women.

Changes in the menstrual cycle

Menstrual cycles become highly variable in regularity and flow. The median length of the cycle shortens from 30 days at 25 years of age to 28 days at 35 years due to a shortened follicular phase. In women with regular periods, the number of anovulatory cycles increases with age.

In the last five to six years before the menopause, only 10% of the cycles are ovulatory.

Immediate and medium-term symptoms

Vasomotor: hot flashes and night sweats Estrogen deficiency symptoms commonly first occur during the perimenopause when ovarian function begins to diminish and hormone levels commonly show wide fluctuations. The most usual estrogen deficiency symptoms are vasomotor symptoms, psychologic symptoms and atrophic changes in estrogen-sensitive tissues. The incidence of vasomotor and psychologic symptoms varies, and in some societies such as Japan it may be only a third of that observed in Western Europe or North America (see Table 3.3).

Table 3.3 Reproductive, health and other differences between North American and Japanese women (Kobe, Kyoto, Nagano – Japan; Manitoba – Canada; Massachusetts – USA)

	Japan	Canada	USA
Surgical menopause*	10	20	30
Menopausal symptoms* (reported in the last 2 weeks)			
hot flashes/sweats	17	46	43
completely asymptomatic	27	14	16
Medicine taking*			
stomach remedy	22	9	11
herbal tea	16	4	3
pain killers	14	45	63
tranquillizers	4	12	10
current HRT use	3	6	8
Breast cancer incidence (per 100 000 women)	23	96	114
CHD deaths (per 100 000)	9.2	34.1	33.5
Hip fracture incidence (per 100 000)	325	788	845

*The numbers shown are percentages of all women in the menopause. HRT, hormone-replacement therapy; CHD, coronary heart disease. Data derived from Kaufert PA, Lock M, McKinlay SM, *et al*. In Lorrain J, ed. *Comprehensive Management of the Menopause*. New York: Springer-Verlag, 1994:59–65

Table 3.4 Non-menopausal causes of hot flashes

Thyrotoxicosis
Carcinoid
Mastocytosis
Anxiety
Diabetes
Pheochromocytoma
Alcohol withdrawal
Epilepsy

SERMS, selective estrogen receptor modulators

Vasomotor symptoms include hot flashes, night sweats, palpitations, headaches and dizziness. In Western countries, 60–75% of women will suffer from hot flashes, which are believed to be a manifestation of hypothalamic thermoregulatory dysfunction. Of these women, 85% will have them for over a year, 25–50% for up to five years and 5% for over 10 years or indefinitely. Hypo-estrogenism *per se* does not strictly speaking cause hot flashes since these are often absent in established postmenopausal women and premenopausal hypo-estrogenic states such as Turner's syndrome, anorexia nervosa and hyperprolactinemia. Rather, it is thought that declining levels of estrogen are responsible for the onset of symptoms.

Interestingly, around 70% of men suffer hot flashes after orchidectomy. Obese women seem to suffer fewer hot flashes, probably due to a greater peripheral conversion of estrogen. However, they can be provoked by alcohol, stress, hot drinks or hot weather. The menopause is not the only cause for hot flashes in middle-aged women and some other, albeit infrequent, causes are listed in Table 3.4.

The hot flash is the subjective sensation of intense warmth in the upper body and typically lasts for 4 min (range 30 s to 5 min). There may be a prodromata of palpitations or headache. The hot flash is frequently accompanied by faintness, weakness or vertigo. The episode ends in profuse sweating and a cold sensation, due to the rise in the cutaneous blood flow followed by a fall in the core body temperature. Hot flashes that happen at night (night sweats) can lead to a reduction of REM (rapid eye movement) sleep with all its consequences, the most important being tiredness, irritability and poor productivity.

Psychologic Over the years a number of psychologic symptoms have been attributed to estrogen deficiency. It is important to recognize that the type of population under study will influence the reporting of psychologic symptoms in the menopausal transition. If the study population consists of women recruited through menopause clinics or advertisements, it is likely that, in this self-selected population, psychologic symptoms will be greater than in the general population of menopausal women. If, however, the study population is unselected, a different picture

Table 3.5 Pre-existing problems that may be accentuated after the menopause

Marital dissatisfaction
Poor health
Financial problems
Bereavement – loss of parent, relative or friend
Severe social stress
   demanding work
   fear of redundancy
Educational/marital difficulties of the children
Aging and/or dependent parents
Lack of social support
Loss of partner (death, separation)
Coming to terms with aging, loss of fertility and
   perceived loss of femininity
Living in youth-oriented society and culture

Table 3.6 The menopause and the genitourinary tract

Vulval/vaginal atrophy
Vaginal dryness
Vaginal infections
Frequency/urgency, dysuria, nocturia
Predisposition to UTIs
Dyspareunia
Decreased libido/frequency of intercourse
Decreased sexual desire
Decreased intensity of orgasm

UTIs, urinary tract infections

appears. The evidence from prospective population-based longitudinal studies suggests that there is no excess of psychologic symptoms during the menopause transition. In particular, in some studies, no direct association between the menopause and depression or psychologic well-being has been found, as well as no increase of anxiety. No clear conclusion has as yet been drawn about cognitive functions and the menopause.

There are a number of pre-existing problems and life changes that occur in middle age (see Table 3.5) and these problems may lead to psychologic symptoms. If, in addition, there are the added problems of hot flashes, night sweats and poor sleep, then the feeling of an inability to cope may develop. The psychologic symptoms may turn into psychologic morbidity, so the menopause may be the straw that breaks the camel's back. It is extremely important that the possibility of this downward spiral is recognized and not allowed to develop. Women should be offered the opportunity to discuss their own perception of their problems and a much wider variety of issues, not just the physical symptoms of the menopause. The treatment should be individualized and may include counseling, psychologic therapy, advice on lifestyle, hormone replacement therapy, antidepressants, or a combination of these.

Genitourinary and sexual Atrophic changes resulting from estrogen deficiency in sensitive connective tissues affect the urogenital tract and, more generally, the skin, hair and nails. Genital tract changes result in atrophic vaginitis, leading to vaginal soreness and dyspareunia. Estrogen deficiency leads to a fall in the number of lactobacilli with an increase of the vaginal pH. The maturation index changes with the number of parabasal cells exceeding the number of superficial cells. Atrophy of the cervix and uterine body and endometrial atrophy occur. The blood flow to the pelvis decreases. The skin generally thins and loses its elasticity and the hair and nails lose their shine and become brittle. Urinary tract changes result in frequency, urgency, dysuria and a predisposition to urinary infections. Changes in sexual function due to the menopause are difficult to disentangle from those related to age. However, it has been reported that intercourse may become painful and less frequent, with orgasm intensity decreased. For a summary of changes in the genitourinary system see Table 3.6.

Long-term effects of the menopause

The long-term effects of the menopause include those on the cardiovascular system, on bone and on other aspects of the metabolism. The long-term consequences are discussed in greater detail in Chapter 6.

Contraception

4

Joanna N. Raeburn, Chris Wilkinson and Nikolai Manassiev

INTRODUCTION

Throughout history, men and women have attempted to control their fertility. The oldest method of contraception in the world is coitus interruptus which, while not being specifically recommended as a method by health professionals, nevertheless remains 'better than nothing' in situations where religious objections or unavailability of other methods of contraception is the only alternative. Apart from coitus interruptus, barrier methods of contraception have been around longest. There is evidence for the use of a form of male condom dating back at least to Roman times, although it is thought that early use of condoms was primarily as a protection against sexually transmitted diseases (STDs) rather than for the prevention of pregnancy. There is also evidence for the use of female barrier methods as long ago as prehistoric Egypt.

In the middle and latter part of the twentieth century, the condom was somewhat eclipsed by the advent of the combined oral contraceptive (COC) pill, but with the spread of HIV infection condoms are once again one of the most widely used methods in the developed world. The great advances of the late twentieth century in terms of human fertility control have been in the development of improved hormonal delivery systems and intrauterine devices (IUDs). Frequency of use of different contraceptive methods in the UK is summarized in Table 4.1.

The effectiveness of various contraceptive methods is measured by means of either the Pearl index or life-table analysis. The Pearl index (named after its inventor, an American biostatistician, and introduced in 1932) is still commonly used, but life-table analysis is more

Table 4.1 Percentage of women aged 15–49 using various methods of contraception

Method	UK
Sterilization	25
Hormonal	23
Condom	16
IUD	5
Abstinence/no partner	16

IUD, intrauterine device

accurate and is gaining in popularity. The Pearl index is calculated from the formula:

Failure rate

$$= \frac{\text{Total accidental pregnancies}}{\text{Total months of exposure}} \times 1200$$

The Pearl index is expressed in terms of a rate of event (i.e., pregnancy) per 100 woman-years. Although suited for scientific studies, the concept of the Pearl index may be difficult for the patient to grasp. In everyday practice it is easier to say that if a failure rate of a contraceptive method is quoted, for example, as 5, it means that if 100 couples use this particular method for one year, five of them will experience failure (pregnancy). The failure rate depends on the efficacy of the method itself (method effectiveness or method failure) and on the ability of the user to use the method correctly (user failure). Some contraceptive users are very careful when using their chosen method (perfect use) and they may be able to achieve a very low failure rate. In case of perfect use the failure rate will be solely due to method failure. However,

Table 4.2 Failure rates for different contraceptive methods

Method	Failure rate range per 100 woman-years
Sterilization	
male	0–0.01
female	0.3–0.5
Implanon (levonorgestrel implant)	0–0.07
Injectables	0.7–0.1
Combined pill (30–35 µg)	0.1–0.4
Progestogen-only pill	0.1–4
IUD (330–380 mm² copper)	0.3–0.6
IUS (Mirena)	< 0.3
Diaphragm	2–15
Condom	2–15
Coitus interruptus	8–17
Fertility awareness	2–26
Spermicides	3–28
Lactational amenorrhea	2–4

IUD, intrauterine device; IUS, intrauterine system

compliance error, intercurrent illness or some other factor may take place which may increase the failure rate (typical use). The failure rate in this case is the sum of method failure and user failure. Because of these considerations the failure rate is often quoted as a range, rather than as a single number. A summary of failure rates for various contraceptive methods is given in Table 4.2. In the USA considerably higher failure rates have been reported for sterilization, injectables and the pill. The effectiveness of contraception by itself does not mean very much unless compared to natural fertility rates. Natural fertility rates vary but the chance of getting pregnant by means of regular unprotected intercourse among unselected couples is about 20–30%, about 60% and about 90% after one, six and 12 months, respectively. There is no reliable figure about the chance of pregnancy after single exposure, but it varies depending on the time of the cycle.

BARRIER METHODS

Male condoms

The male condom is the cheapest and most readily available method of contraception worldwide; it needs no intervention from health professionals, has no adverse health effects on the user and confers undoubted health benefits on both partners. With careful use, condoms can be an extremely effective method of contraception, with the additional benefit of protection against sexually transmitted infections (STIs). Failure rates are quoted as between 2 and 15% per annum, the difference relating to that between 'perfect' use and 'typical' use. All users of condoms should be aware of the availability and limitations of emergency contraception in case of condom failure, but sadly many condom accidents go unnoticed by the users and result in unintended pregnancies. Most condoms available in the UK are made of latex rubber. Latex allergy occasionally occurs and condoms made of polyurethane have been developed. Both types of condom have their benefits and drawbacks; latex condoms may be weakened or damaged by oil-based lubricants, including such commonly used substances as Vaseline, baby oil, edible creams and certain medicinal products such as several anti-candidal preparations and estrogen creams and pessaries. Polyurethane condoms are not affected by these products and also have better storage life than latex condoms. However, in normal use latex condoms have lower breakage rates and lower slippage and failure rates than polyurethane condoms, and the latter are probably best reserved for those couples suffering from latex allergy.

Practical advice

The best way to teach condom usage is with a plastic condom demonstrator; the principal points that need to be made are as follows:

(1) Condoms are for single use only.

(2) Avoid any mechanical damage, e.g., from sharp fingernails when the condom is being handled.

(3) Space needs to be left at the tip of the condom for the ejaculate; this is normally provided by the manufacturer in the

form of a small teat, which should be emptied of air prior to application.

(4) The condom should be unrolled only when placed over the tip of the erect penis and must be put on the right way round so that the rolled-up rim can be easily rolled down the shaft of the penis.

(5) No genital contact should take place before the condom is put on.

(6) The rim of the condom must be held firmly at the time of withdrawal, to prevent the condom slipping off.

(7) Oil-based lubricants should be avoided when using latex condoms; water-based lubricants such as KY jelly or a spermicidal gel should be advised instead.

Non-contraceptive benefits of condoms

Latex condoms reduce the incidence of STIs. This is particularly so with bacterial infections such as gonorrhea but reductions in the risk of transmitting chlamydia and trichomoniasis have also been observed. Additionally, there is significant protection against the blood-borne viruses HIV and hepatitis B and C, but less in the case of conditions that may affect the vulva and shaft of penis, such as wart and herpes viruses.

In addition, there is evidence that regular use of condoms leads to a lower risk of cervical intraepithelial neoplasia. For many women, particularly younger ones who may not yet be in permanent monogamous relationships, the use of condoms is recommended as additional protection in conjunction with hormonal or intrauterine methods of contraception – the so-called 'Double Dutch' method providing effective contraception combined with protection against STDs.

Diaphragms and cervical caps

Vaginal barrier methods have been in use throughout the last century but their popularity has sharply declined since the immediate pre-pill era in the 1950s, when they were the

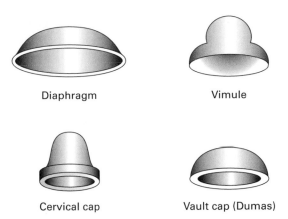

Diaphragm

Vimule

Cervical cap

Vault cap (Dumas)

Figure 4.1 Female barrier devices: diaphragm and cervical caps

principal method of contraception available to women. Nowadays, the most commonly used vaginal barrier is the diaphragm (originally known as the 'Dutch cap') (Figure 4.1). In the UK, the diaphragm is often popularly referred to as 'the cap' and in our further discussion these terms are used interchangeably. Other barriers such as the cervical cap, the Vimule and the vault or Dumas cap (Figure 4.1) are rarely used or available nowadays. They may have an occasional place for women who have difficulties with placement of diaphragms or recurrent cystitis.

The diaphragm has the advantage over the condom in that firstly it is under the woman's control, and secondly it can be inserted well before intercourse and need not therefore interrupt the spontaneity of the sex. It does not, however, confer the same degree of protection against STIs as does the condom, although regular users of vaginal barriers are at lower risk of cervical neoplasia and pelvic infection.

The efficacy of the diaphragm varies according to user motivation and consistency of use but failure rates between 4 and 18% per annum are quoted. Undoubtedly, though, before the advent of hormonal methods of contraception, let alone emergency contraception, there were families throughout the developed world whose size was arrived at not by accident but by careful use of the Dutch cap throughout the fertile years. In recent years, a number of new vaginal barrier methods have been developed. These include the female condom or Femidom, the 'sponge', Femcap and the disposable Oves cervical cap, which can stay in place for three days.

Types of diaphragm

The diaphragm is a thin circular dome-shaped piece of rubber, edged with a rubber-coated metal rim. The external diameter of the rim is the size of the diaphragm, changing in increments of 5 mm. The size range is 50–105 mm, the most widely used sizes being 65–80 mm. The diaphragm fits between the posterior vaginal fornix and behind the pubic symphysis (Figure 4.2), thus covering the cervix and isolating it from penile contact. Three types of diaphragm are currently available: flat spring, coil spring and arcing spring. Flat spring diaphragms have a firmer feel to the rim than coil spring ones: consequently many women find the latter more comfortable in use. Arcing spring diaphragms are more expensive than the other types, and combine features of both; when squeezed prior to insertion in the vagina, they form a curved arch shape which helps to direct the diaphragm into the right position with the leading edge in the posterior fornix. This is an advantage for women who find it difficult to insert a flat or coil spring diaphragm over an awkwardly placed cervix. In women with poor vaginal muscle tone, a cystocoele or a rectocoele, the cervical cap may prove more appropriate as its correct use is independent of vaginal tone.

Advice to patients

The successful use of vaginal barriers requires careful initial assessment and fitting by a trained health professional. A correctly sized and fitted diaphragm should be comfortable to the wearer to the extent that she should not be aware of its presence either before, during or after intercourse; neither should it interfere with her partner's sensations (although he may be able to feel it). The size of the diaphragm is

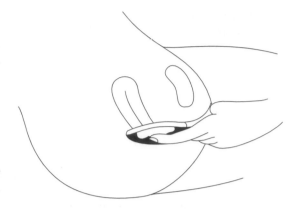

Figure 4.2 Insertion of the diaphragm. Reproduced with permission from Kleinman RL, ed. *Family Planning Handbook for Doctors*. London: International Planned Parenthood Federation, 1988:135

determined by vaginal examination and is taken as the distance from the tip of the index finger placed in the posterior fornix to the interior rim of the pubic arch. This is not an exact science and, in practice, there is no single size that fits an individual woman. The size of diaphragm chosen may vary between equally experienced health professionals, according to whether a very tight fit behind the pubic arch or a smaller device simply covering the cervix is preferred. The use of spermicides with any vaginal barrier is always recommended and women requesting 'cap fitting' should be shown how to apply spermicidal jelly and how to insert and remove the cap. It is generally good practice to send the woman away with the cap to practice for a week, relying on an alternative method of contraception in the meantime. At the return visit, with the cap in place, its fit and correct placement covering the cervix can be checked and, if all is well, the woman can then rely on it as her method of contraception.

Practical considerations

(1) The cap should not be inserted more than 2 h before intercourse; if over 2 h have elapsed without intercourse taking place, it should be removed, further spermicide applied and reinserted.

(2) Following sexual intercourse, the cap should be left in place for a minimum of 6 h and a maximum of 24 h.

(3) If intercourse is repeated during the 6 h period, the cap should be left in place but further spermicide added, either by using an applicator to apply cream or jelly or by use of a pessary inserted high in the vagina next to the cap.

(4) The cap can be inserted either way up but some spermicide should be in contact with the cervix; additional spermicide can be placed around the rim of the cap to lubricate and thus aid insertion.

It is traditionally recommended that the size of a cap should be checked after childbirth and after gain or loss of more than 3 kg in weight; in practice it is not common for the size to change significantly and, as stated earlier, there is no 'one and only' correct size at any one time. The woman herself is probably the best judge of whether her cap is the right size, as a cap that is too large will be uncomfortable and will not sit correctly behind the pubic symphysis, while a cap that is too small will feel loose and will frequently be difficult to remove.

Other female barrier methods

The Femidom, or female condom (Figure 4.3), is made of lubricated polyurethane and resembles a small plastic pouch with two soft rings, one at either end. The purpose of the rings is to assist placement of the Femidom, the inner ring at the closed end of the pouch being guided toward the cervix, while the outer ring, at the open end of the pouch, is placed outside the vagina over the labias. As it covers a greater area of the female genitalia, it is potentially a superior barrier to STIs than male condoms but there are no reliable data to support this assertion. Although the Femidom is not widely used in the UK it should not be dismissed without discussion because the method does suit some couples.

The Today sponge, which was essentially a vehicle for spermicide rather than a barrier

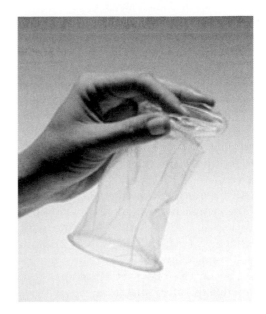

Figure 4.3 Female condom. Reproduced with permission from The Female Health Company, UK

method, is no longer available in the UK; its high failure rate made it only really suitable for women requiring 'spacing' contraception or in those women whose fertility is exceedingly low anyway (see below, under 'Spermicides').

The Oves cap is a single-use silicone cervical cap, which can be left in place for up to 72 h but must not be used during menstruation. Like other types of vaginal barrier, it is recommended to be used with a spermicide. It is available from some pharmacies but women are advised to see their family planning provider to fit the right size and train the woman in its use.

Spermicides

In general, spermicides alone are not recommended as a reliable method of contraception, as their failure rate ranges from 3 to 28%. Spermicides should be used in conjunction with diaphragms and cervical caps. In perimenopausal women, particularly where the menstrual cycle appears to have ceased and symptoms of estrogen deficiency, such as hot flashes, are beginning to appear, a spermicidal foam or pessary may provide adequate cover. If aged under 50 years, women are advised to continue with contraceptive precautions for two years after the last menstrual period (LMP), and if over 50, for one year after the LMP. In all other age groups, the use of spermicides alone should be discouraged and they should always be combined with a barrier method such as described above.

All spermicides available in the UK contain as the active ingredient nonoxynol-9, combined with a surfactant to aid spread in the vagina and a gel or cream carrier compound. They are available as gels, creams, foams and also pessaries. The first three are effective immediately after insertion while pessaries need 10 minutes to dissolve before intercourse takes place. All spermicides remain active in the vagina for a maximum of 2 h.

Spermicides such as nonoxynol-9 and other related compounds have been shown *in vitro* to have microbicidal activity and are active against several sexually transmitted organisms, including chlamydia, gonococcus and trichomonas. They do not, however, provide full protection against these infections *in vivo*, and there is doubt as to whether they are effective as viricides. It is also suspected that spermicides, when used very frequently, lead to inflammation of the vaginal epithelium which may in turn increase the likelihood of viral transmission – such as HIV.

NATURAL FAMILY PLANNING

Natural family planning (also known as periodic abstinence) can be a successful method of contraception, although widely varying failure rates, between 2 and 26%, are quoted. The greater level of success is only achieved with fairly intensive training by an experienced teacher of the method – usually, but not invariably, a specially trained family planning nurse; and by a very high degree of commitment and self-control on the part of the couple.

The method relies on identifying the fertile phase of the menstrual cycle and avoiding intercourse until the phase is over. There are a number of indicators of fertile and infertile phases of the cycle, which can be learnt and used to identify safe and unsafe times for sexual intercourse, depending on whether pregnancy is sought or is to be avoided. The so-called 'major indicators' are changes in the quality and quantity of cervical mucus, the position of the cervix and the basal body temperature (BBT). Minor indicators, such as ovulation pain ('Mittelschmerz'), mid-cycle bleeding and breast pain, which may be readily recognizable by some women, may also contribute to the calculation. For successful natural family planning it is recommended that women rely on at least two – and preferably three – major indicators.

Mucus changes

For most of the cycle the cervical mucus is either absent or scanty, and thick, while in the immediate pre-ovulation phase the mucus becomes profuse, thin and stretchy (Spinnbarkeit, Figure 4.4), frequently being described as resembling raw egg white. Properties of the cervical mucus are also discussed in Chapter 1. These differences can be detected by the woman who examines her mucus on a regular basis and indicate the fertile period immediately leading up to ovulation, when intercourse should be avoided by those not wishing to conceive. One has to bear in mind that changes in cervical mucus can be masked by seminal fluids, spermicides or vaginal infection.

Changes in the cervix

During the fertile phase, the cervix rises higher in the vagina and the os becomes slightly more open, whilst at other times of the cycle the cervix is lower in the vagina and the os feels tightly closed. Again, these changes can be recognized by those who examine themselves

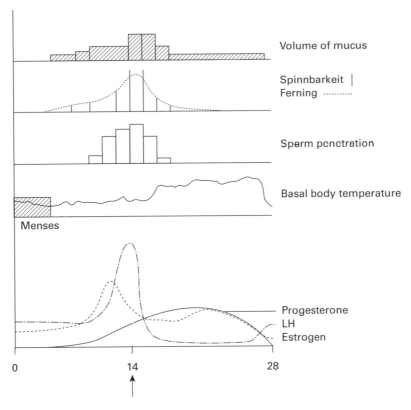

Figure 4.4 Changes in cervical mucus and basal body temperature in relation to the menstrual cycle. Reproduced with permission from Johnson MH, Everitt BJ. *Essential Reproduction*, 2nd edn. Oxford: Blackwell Scientific Publishers, 1984:171

regularly and can contribute to knowledge of the fertile phase.

Basal body temperature

The progesterone surge produced at the time of ovulation leads to a small rise in BBT of between 0.2 and 0.6°C and the temperature remains at this higher level until the onset of menstruation (Figure 4.4). The woman should be instructed to take her temperature each morning before rising, using a special 'fertility thermometer', which is widely graduated over a narrow temperature range to facilitate recognition of small differences in temperature. The temperature rise indicates

that ovulation has taken place and, therefore, it has no place as a predictor of ovulation. Once the temperature rise has been detected for three consecutive mornings, ovulation can be considered over, the ovum no longer viable and intercourse can take place without protection.

From the above it can readily be seen that more than one indicator is needed, simply because the mucus and cervical changes indicate the onset of the fertile phase, while the BBT is an indicator of the end of the fertile phase. In practice, the mucus changes are not always as clear as described, particularly if the woman is combining natural family planning with a barrier method of contraception for the 'unsafe' times. The BBT changes can be obscured by many factors, including stress, disturbed nights, fever and alcohol, while some women cannot easily recognize the cervical changes.

Fertility monitors

New developments to try and bring science to the aid of the determined natural family planner include the 'Persona' monitor. This device monitors the changes in levels of urinary luteinizing hormone (LH) and estrogen metabolites to indicate the start and finish of the fertile phase. It is *not* recommended for women who have a cycle length outside a 23–35 days' range, are perimenopausal, have polycystic ovarian syndrome have liver or kidney diseases or are breastfeeding. The efficacy of Persona can be reduced by medications that alter LH and estrogen metabolism, and the manufacturer's instructions should be followed. The Persona system has a quoted failure rate of about 6% for perfect use, which is higher than many women are prepared to accept. However, it is non-invasive, does not have side-effects, is easy to use and may appeal to couples keen to practice natural family planning. It is not available on the NHS.

Lactational amenorrhea method

In the developing world, anovulation and amenorrhea associated with full breastfeeding is the principal method of contraception. It appears that pulsatile secretion of gonadotropin-releasing hormone (GnRH) is suppressed by infant suckling (via prolactin), which leads to suppression of release of LH; this in turn causes failure of follicular development and thus of ovulation. For this to occur, it is important that the infant should be fully breastfed, without supplements, on demand, including during the night. If supplements are given, they should only be given after the infant has been breastfed to maintain the maximal suckling stimulus.

The lactational amenorrhea method (LAM) is defined as follows:

(1) The woman is fully breastfeeding, day and night, with few supplements;

(2) The woman is amenorrheic;

(3) The infant is less than six months old.

If a patient fulfills all three of the above criteria, she can be advised that her contraceptive protection is approximately 98% and that this efficacy is comparable to other methods of contraception available in the postpartum period. In those rural parts of the world where women traditionally breastfeed for prolonged periods and access to health care and family planning services may be limited, LAM may be extended. For example, in Rwanda a program entitled LAM-9 was introduced in which there was good efficacy up to nine months postpartum without the use of any additional contraceptive method. In the developed world, where food supplements are frequently introduced well before the infant is six months old, it may be advisable to introduce additional contraceptive methods at around three to four months.

HORMONAL CONTRACEPTION

An increasingly expanding variety of hormonal contraception is now available to women. The common feature of all of these agents is that synthetic estrogenic and/or progestogenic compounds are used in order to suppress ovulation and change the endometrium, cervical mucus and tubal motility in order to prevent pregnancy. The expansion of hormonal contraception is due to (1) the number of chemical compounds being available; (2) various dosages; and (3) routes of administration. In our discussion of hormonal contraception, we shall touch on transdermal and vaginal routes, on a new progestogen (drospirene) as well as on the first progestogen-only pill that reliably suppresses ovulation.

Combined oral contraceptives

The development of the combined oral contraceptive (COC) pill in the late 1950s was the start of a revolution in women's reproductive health care. For the first time, women had a reliable method of contraception that was independent of intercourse. The original pill contained, by today's standards, huge quantities of the synthetic progestogen, norethynodrel, and the estrogen, mestranol. Although 'the pill', as the combined contraceptive pill came to be known, has been the subject of more investigation than probably any other medicine in the twentieth century, only one randomized prospective study of pill use, compared with a barrier method, has ever been performed. This was carried out in Puerto Rico, with recruitment of nearly 10 000 women between 1960 and 1969, who were followed up until the trial was abandoned in 1976. Due to the long duration of the study, there were very high drop-out rates during the follow-up period and also switching of contraceptive methods between groups.

These early studies appeared to show no significant health differences between pill users and non-users, despite the fact that the doses of synthetic hormones in the pill at that time were vastly higher than are used nowadays. However, our understanding of the risks and benefits of the COC pill has been refined as the quality of research has improved. The Royal College of General Practitioners' (RCGP) study, for example, carried out in the late 1960s and early 1970s looked at, amongst other things, the incidence and type of vascular disease in pill users, and it was studies like this which first demonstrated the association between pill use and venous thromboembolism (VTE). The RCGP study was also based on pills containing much higher doses of estrogen and progestogen than are in current use because it was not until 1974 that pills containing 30 or 35 μg of the estrogen ethinylestradiol (EE) were introduced. The development of low-dose (30 and 35 μg/day) COCs was initiated as a result of these studies, which had suggested that some of the observed adverse effects might be related to the amount of estrogen. In addition, there has been a progressive trend toward reducing both the dose and the potency of the progestogen content of the pill, with the result that all studies relating to higher-dose pills must be interpreted with caution when considering the present-day pill user and her potential risks.

Classification of combined oral contraceptives

There are three main ways of categorizing COCs: by dose (amount of estrogen), by generation (type of estrogen and progestogen), and by variation in dose (phasic pills) (see Figure 4.5 and Appendix I).

Dose High-dose pills contain 50 μg/day EE or more; in the UK Ovran and norinyl-1 are the only high-dose COC licensed and are used only for women on hepatic enzyme-inducing drugs. Low-dose pills contain 30–35 μg/day EE and constitute the majority of COCs in current use in the UK. Ultra-low dose pills are those with less than 30 μg/day EE. They are not widely used and, whilst maintaining contraceptive efficacy, tend to be associated with increased breakthrough bleeding. It is likely that ultra-low dose pills will be refined in time and become more widely used.

Generation Three generations of pills are currently described:

(1) First-generation pills are no longer available. They all contained 50 μg of EE or more. The original estrogen was mestranol, which is the pro-drug of EE, and this was combined with progestogens that are no longer in use in combined preparations, such as lynoestrenol and ethynodiol diacetate. Brand names included Minovlar, very widely used in the early 1970s, and Minilyn and Conova 30, both of which were still available in the early 1990s.

(2) Second-generation pills are currently the most widely used. They include the pills containing 30–35 μg/day of EE in

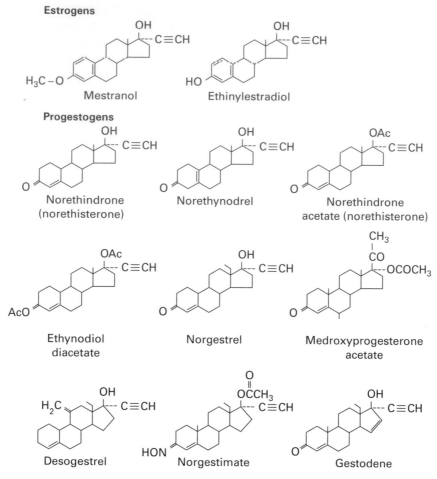

Figure 4.5 Some synthetic estrogens and progestogens used in hormonal methods of contraception

combination with one of the following progestogens: norethisterone, norethisterone acetate and levonorgestrel. Included in this group are the very widely prescribed Microgynon/Ovranette and Ovysmen/Brevinor.

(3) Third-generation pills contain 20–30 μg/day EE and the progestogens gestodene or desogestrel. These exhibit less androgenic side-effects than the second-generation progestogens. The branded names are Femodene/Minulet and Marvelon/Mercilon. Preparations containing the progestogen norgestimate are usu- ally regarded as third-generation pills. However, norgestimate is a pro-drug for levonorgestrel which is a second-generation progestogen.

(4) Efforts continue to improve the metabolic effects and tolerability of the current progestogens. Some such progestogens are: dienogest, drospirenone, nestorone, nomegestrol and trimegestone. Dienogest is licensed in Germany in COC pill and hormone replacement therapy formulations. Trimegestone is available in France. The combination of drospirenone and EE is licensed in the UK as the COC pill

Yasmin. The properties of drospirenone are such that Yasmin cannot be classified as either second- or third-generation COC. Drospirenone is discussed further below.

Phasic pills   Monophasic pills have a constant dose of EE and progestogen throughout the 21-day course of pills. Triphasic pills attempt to mimic the natural menstrual cycle by varying the doses of both EE and progestogen over the course of 21 days of pill taking. Biphasic pills have been developed but there are no biphasic pills available in the UK at the time of writing. In general, bi- and triphasic pills appear to offer no significant advantages over monophasic pills, although, on an individual basis, they may suit some women better.

Efficacy, mechanism of action and metabolic effects of the pill

The contraceptive efficacy of COCs is generally quoted as between 0.1 and 0.4 pregnancies per 100 woman-years; this is with perfect use. The actual failure rate varies in practice according to the compliance of the user and the length of time of use. The Oxford Family Planning Association contraceptive study reported a failure rate of 0.2 per 100 woman-years, but US data suggests a failure rate of 5–7% during the first 12 months of use. The main mechanism of action of COCs is by inhibition of the normal secretion of LH and follicle-stimulating hormone (FSH) from the pituitary and this results in inhibition of ovulation. The three additional mechanisms are: (1) thickening of the cervical mucus leading to reduced sperm penetration; (2) development of endometrial changes making it less receptive to implantation of the blastocyst; and (3) changes in the motility (reduced) and secretion of the fallopian tubes. Ovulation is suppressed if at the beginning of the cycle seven pills are taken consecutively. If two or more pills are missed from the first seven of the pack, or four or more pills are missed from the middle of the pack, then ovulation may arise.

The use of synthetic sex steroids leads to a number of metabolic changes. Some of them are of scientific interest only but others (coagulation, lipids, etc.) may be of considerable clinical significance (see Table 4.3). Second- and third-generation COCs show differences with regard to certain metabolic characteristics. Third-generation COCs seem to affect coagulation more than second-generation COCs, and users of third-generation COCs have a higher risk of VTE than users of second-generation COCs. However, users of third-generation COCs seem to have a lower risk of myocardial infarction in comparison with the second-generation users. The picture is bound to become more complicated with the introduction of drospirenone in Yasmin. Each Yasmin pill contains 30 µg EE and 3 mg drospirenone. Drospirenone is a derivative of spironolactone and has mild antimineral corticoid activity and anti-androgenic activity. One metabolic study comparing Yasmin with Microgynon showed that in Yasmin users the systolic blood pressure decreased by 2.9 mmHg and the diastolic blood pressure by 3.4 mmHg, high-density lipoprotein and triglyceride levels increased and low-denisity lipoprotein levels fell; there was no change in glucose tolerance. Whether these changes are of any clinical significance is not yet known. Yasmin apart, in general, there is a small increase in the blood pressure that is of no clinical significance in most women (the increase is in the range of 7–8 mmHg for systolic blood pressure and 5–6 mmHg for diastolic blood pressure). However, regular blood pressure monitoring is very important to identify the small minority of women who may develop clinically significant hypertension.

Key history, indications and contraindications for combined oral contraceptives

Medical and family history   As with any other area of medicine, good contraceptive care requires careful history taking. All methods of contraception are safe, but for some women there are situations where the risk of complications or failure increases. Relevant changes in medical or surgical history may mean that

Table 4.3 Metabolic changes associated with the pill

Coagulation*	Increase in factors II, VII, VIII, IX, X. Decrease in antithrombin and factor V
Lipids*	Increase in total cholesterol and triglycerides. Slight decrease in HDL-cholesterol
Endocrine system	Increase in insulin, adrenal steroids, thyroxin and prolactin*. Decrease in LH, FSH, endogenous estrogen and progesterone. Increase in plasma renin activity and aldosterone secretion
Liver	Increased synthesis of α-2 globulin. Production of more lithogenic bile*
Carbohydrate metabolism	Increased insulin resistance

*Denotes changes of clinical significance; HDL, high-density liproprotein; LH, luteinizing hormone; FSH, follicle-stimulating hormone

use of COCs is partially or completely contraindicated. It is the responsibility of the doctor or nurse providing contraceptive care to take a relevant personal medical and family history (Table 4.4) and to inform patients when the risks for them are different from the norm. As both the medical and family history may change, it is important to review the relevant history at each follow-up visit.

With regard to COCs, the most important areas of history to be considered are those relating to vascular disease. Coronary heart disease (CHD), cerebrovascular disease and VTE are very rare in the majority of young women including those who take COCs; however, in the presence of risk factors (see Table 4.5) this situation can be very different. The effect of risk factors on the hazards associated with COC use is discussed later in this section. In general, the presence of one risk factor is regarded as a relative contraindication and the presence of two summates to become an absolute contraindication to COC use. It is important to remember that common factors such as smoking and obesity constitute arterial disease risks. Migraine is a recognized risk factor for ischemic stroke. In the presence of focal neurologic symptoms preceding the onset of headache and known as aura, these risks are increased further and COCs are contraindicated, usually for life. The diagnosis of migraine with or without

Table 4.4 Relevant family history in first-degree relatives to be taken before prescribing combined oral contraceptives

Venous thromboembolism and embolism

Early onset cardiovascular disease < 50 years, including
  angina
  myocardial infarction
  hypertension
  stroke
  hyperlipidemia
  carcinoma of the breast

Hyperlipidemia

Carcinoma of the breast

aura is made on basis of the history and the absence of other neurologic disease. The diagnosis is usually clear but when atypical a neurologic referral may be required to support the diagnosis of migraine. Sickle cell disease was previously regarded as a contraindication to COCs because of the risk of thrombosis during crises. Whilst COC is not a first-line method (Depo-Provera is associated with a reduction in the frequency of crises), its use appears to be safe and it is widely used in these patients as the risk of sickle cell disease in pregnancy and associated complications far outweighs the risk of COC use; however, in the authors' opinion it is not recommendable in a patient suffering from frequent sickle crises.

Table 4.5 Risk factors for cardiovascular disease

Venous disease risk factors

(1) Personal history of VTE[*]
(2) Known thrombophilia
(3) Severe varicose veins
(4) Immobility, e.g., bed-bound
(5) History of VTE occurring in first-degree relative
(6) History of thrombophilia in close relative

Arterial disease risk factors

(1) Known arterial disease
(2) Age > 35
(3) Current smoking (especially > 20 per day) or ex-smoker within six months of stopping
(4) Hypertension[†]
(5) Migraine (risk factor for ischemic stroke)
(6) Hyperlipidemia/familial hyperlipidemia
(7) Diabetes
(8) Family history of arterial disease (ischemic heart disease, strokes), especially occurring < 50 years old or of familial hyperlipidemia
(9) Obesity

[*]Does not include phlebitis, an inflammation of the superficial veins, which according to a number of respected journals and societies is not a risk factor for venous thromboembolism (VTE)
[†]Uncontrolled hypertension is an absolute contraindication to combined oral contraceptive (COC) use; in cases of controlled hypertension without any other additional risk factor COCs can be used with caution

A history of hormone-dependent conditions, such as pemphigoid gestationis, cholestatic jaundice of pregnancy, certain types of porphyria or chloasma (this is not an absolute contraindication), may contraindicate COC use. A personal and family history of breast cancer should be noted because there is an increased risk of having breast cancer diagnosed whilst taking COCs, compared to never users (for more detail see page 52). Women with a strong family history of carcinoma of the breast can use COCs, but only after having all the potential ramifications explained, and they may need referral to a breast clinic for further advice. Current, active liver disease or elevated liver-function tests within the previous three months is a contraindication to COC use.

Drug history/interactions Older anticonvulsants such as phenytoin, carbamazepine and phenobarbitone, griseofulvin and certain anti-HIV drugs, all of which act as liver enzyme inducers, cause reduced contraceptive efficacy as a result of increased metabolism of both the estrogen and progestogen. If COCs are to be used, patients should be treated with a 50 µg estrogen pill, possibly with a decreased pill-free interval or tricycling (three packets taken without a break), throughout the treatment and for up to 4 weeks after stopping it. Newer anticonvulsants, such as sodium valproate, gabapentin and lamotrigine, do not have this effect. Rifampicin and rifabutin are such powerful enzyme inducers that alternative contraceptives should be used. Particular care should be taken when short courses of rifampicin are used as prophylaxis following close contact with meningococcal meningitis. Even just two days of treatment can lead to decreased contraceptive efficacy for up to four weeks, and patients must be properly advised if pregnancy is to be avoided as well as an outbreak of meningitis.

Gynecologic history Prescribers should enquire about the menstrual cycle, in particular its regularity, the cycle length, menstrual loss, and about the presence of dysmenorrhea and premenstrual problems. Enquiry should be made as to whether there have been prior episodes of amenorrhea not caused by pregnancy. Contraceptive history should be noted, in particular the reasons for discontinuing any previously used methods.

Social history It is important in all age groups to take a smoking history, although smoking will not be regarded as an absolute contraindication to COC use in women under 35 years of age unless it is associated with other cardiovascular risk factors. However, no opportunity should be lost for life-style advice, and young women should be helped and encouraged to give up smoking as early as possible.

Indications The history can also identify conditions that may be indications for COCs or that may benefit from COCs such as menorrhagia, dysmenorrhea, uterine fibroids, acne, polycystic ovarian syndrome, recurrent functional ovarian cysts and premenstrual syndrome (see Non-contraceptive benefits on this page).

Contraindications These can be divided into absolute and relative contraindications to the COC pill, and are summarized in Tables 4.6 and 4.7.

Wherever a relative contraindication to prescribing is encountered, a balance must be sought between the potential risk of prescribing COCs and both the potential risk of pregnancy to a patient left unprotected, and unwilling or unable to use alternative methods of contraception, and the known non-contraceptive benefits of COCs.

Non-contraceptive benefits

In any discussion of the risks and benefits of COC use, it is very important to convey the many non-contraceptive benefits which are not widely appreciated by the lay public. Established benefits include a very substantial reduction in menorrhagia, with consequent reductions in iron-deficiency anemia. It should be noted that the most common cause of anemia in the reproductive age is menorrhagia. Another benefit is relief of dysmenorrhea. There is a reduced incidence of both benign breast and ovarian disease, with fewer functional ovarian cysts, due to the prevention of ovulation and a reduction in the incidence of pelvic inflammatory disease (PID). Perhaps of most importance, particularly in the light of anxieties about possible increased risk of carcinoma of the breast, is the evidence that COCs offer protection against both endometrial and ovarian carcinoma. Specifically, there appears to be an approximately 40% reduction in risk of ovarian cancer in ever users, this effect being apparent after just one year of use, with greater protection with increased durations of use, and with the effect persisting for up to 15 years after stopping COCs. With endometrial cancer, the reduction in risk appears after two years' use of COCs and persists for up to 10 years after stopping the pill.

COCs have a place in the management of acne in young women, with improvements in this skin condition with several different preparations. The best is Dianette, which contains 35 μg/day of EE and 2 mg/day of cyproterone acetate. This is not licensed in the UK as a contraceptive but is safe and effective for this purpose. On the minus side is the fact that the risk of non-fatal and fatal VTE with the EE/cyproterone combination is higher than with a third-generation COC. Once the acne and/or hirsutism has resolved, the manufacturer advises to stop the treatment. EE/norgestimate (Cilest) is also effective against acne and probably the safer option. Other potential benefits of COCs are a possible role in the prevention of osteoporosis in women and some emerging evidence of a protective effect against rheumatoid arthritis, although results of studies are not entirely consistent and further research in this area is required. A summary of the health benefits of COCs is given in Table 4.8.

Table 4.6   Absolute contraindications to combined oral contraceptives (COC)

Cardiovascular	Severe hypertension > 160/100
	Ischemic heart disease
	Migraine with aura/transient cerebral ischemia
	Personal history of VTE
	Known thrombophilia
	Elective major surgery within next 4 weeks
Diabetes mellitus	Only if microvascular complications present, > 35 years old, smoker, hypertensive
Impaired liver function	Active hepatitis
	Cholestatic jaundice of pregnancy
	Liver tumors
	Dubin–Johnson or Rotor syndromes
Hormone-dependent tumor	Breast cancer or hormone-dependent tumor (although if COC is the only acceptable and suitable method of contraception its use may be considered in discussion with the patient and her oncologist)
	Trophoblastic disease (until serum hCG undetectable)
History of serious conditions related to sex steroids	Porphyria
	Pemphigoid gestationis
	Hemolytic uremic syndrome
Smoking	If over age 35
Severe obesity	BMI $\geq$ 40 kg/m^2
Women over 35 years	In association with:
	(1) Smoking
	(2) Obesity
	(3) Hypertension
	(4) Diabetes
	(5) Familial hyperlipidemia

VTE, venous thromboembolism; hCG, human chorionic gonadotropin; BMI, body mass index

Health risks of combined oral contraceptives in perspective

Myocardial infarction   Myocardial infarction, both fatal and non-fatal, is a very rare event in young women of reproductive age and in non-smoking women under the age of 35. For the everyday practice age, hypertension, smoking, obesity and diabetes are the major risk factors for myocardial infarction and the risk is potentiated by COC use. The case fatality rate for myocardial infarction in pill users is 30%. In a woman with no cardiovascular risk factors, use of the combined pill leads to little or no increase in cardiovascular risk.

In summary (see Table 4.9):

(1)   Serious cardiovascular risks are very low in non-smoking women under the age of 35 with no cardiovascular risk factors.

(2)   In healthy women with no risk factors COC use increases the risk of myocardial infarction by 1–2.5-fold depending on age.

Table 4.7 Relative contraindications to combined oral contraceptives (COCs)

Cardiovascular	Family history of VTE
	Family history of premature arterial cardiovascular disease
	Mild hypertension > 140/90 but < 160/100
Obesity	BMI ≥ 30 kg/m²
Migraine	Simple migraine without aura
Smoker of any age	> 20 cigarettes per day
Puerperal psychosis	
Lactation	
Undiagnosed menstrual abnormality	COCs can be prescribed after appropriate investigations carried out and pelvic pathology excluded
Undiagnosed second-degree amenorrhea	As above

VTE, venous thromboembolism; BMI, body mass index

Table 4.8 Benefits of combined oral contraceptives

Condition	Risk reduction (%)
Pregnancy	> 99
Ectopic pregnancy	90
Functional ovarian cysts	65
Pelvic inflammatory disease	50
Menorrhagia	50
Iron deficiency	50
Dysmenorrhea	50
Primary infertility	40
Ovarian cancer	40–50
Endometrial cancer	40–50
Benign breast disease	40
Acne	Variable

Table 4.9 Absolute risk of myocardial infarction per 10^6 women per annum

	Under 35	Over 35
Non-smoker, no COCs	< 1	12
Non-smoker on COCs	< 4	40
Smoker, no COCs	8	85
Smoker on COCs	40	485

COC, combined oral contraceptive

(3) Smoking increases the relative risk of myocardial infarction five- to ten-fold, depending on the number of cigarettes smoked.

(4) Hypertension increases the risk five- to six-fold.

(5) Obesity (body mass index (BMI) > 30) and diabetes increase the risk three- to four-fold.

Stroke Cerebrovascular accidents are rare in young women of reproductive age; they may occur as the result of ischemia or hemorrhage. Significant risk factors for both ischemic and hemorrhagic stroke are age, hypertension and smoking, while migraine is a risk factor for ischemic stroke only. There appears to be a small increase in relative risk (RR = 2) of ischemic stroke in women using COCs, compared to non-users, but this must be taken in the context of the low background risk. In contrast, there is no increase in risk for hemorrhagic stroke, in women under 35, using COCs without any of the above risk factors. For both ischemic and hemorrhagic stroke, there is no evidence of increased risk with increasing duration of use, nor is there any past use effect. The data regarding the pill and ischemic stroke are summarized in Table 4.10. The case fatality rate for ischemic stroke is 25%.

Venous thromboembolism Despite being the commonest cardiovascular event in COC users, the absolute risk of VTE remains low. In 1995, the Committee on Safety of Medicines advised doctors that there was a significant difference between second- and third-generation COCs with respect to risk of venous thrombosis. Although the data were in fact good news because they suggested that the risk of VTE with the second-generation pill was less (15 per 100 000) than previously thought (40 per 100 000), they were taken as being bad news. This led to many women stopping COC. The difference between the COC generations and VTE has been much debated both for its biologic plausibility and the reliability of the data used, and new revised risks were published in 1999 (see Table 4.11). No difference in the incidence of arterial disease has been observed between second- and third-generation COCs.

The differences between second- and third-generation pills do not justify changing the prescriptions of established pill users. However, all pill users should have the risks explained to them in terms that they are able to understand, with emphasis on the difference between relative and absolute risks. In the case of first-time pill users, it is good clinical practice to commence patients on second-generation pills. They do carry a lower VTE risk and it seems sensible to take the safest option. It is not routine policy in the UK to screen new pill users for coagulation disorders in the absence of a family history of thrombophilia. If a second-generation pill is not tolerated for any reason, then it is perfectly acceptable to change to a third-generation pill.

Where a family history of VTE exists in a first- or even second-degree relative, some recommend screening for hereditary thrombophilias may be indicated. Such screens look for Factor V Leiden mutations (5% prevalence in Caucasians), protein C, protein S and antithrombin deficiencies (combined prevalence of 1–2%) and mutations in the prothrombin gene 20210 (2–4% prevalence in Caucasians). One of the most well studied abnormalities,

Table 4.10 Absolute and relative risk of ischemic stroke per 100 000 women per annum

Background risk	4.4 (RR = 1)
Women with migraine	12 (RR = 3–8)
COC users, no migraine	9.0 (RR = 2)
COC users with migraine	22 (RR = 5)
COC users and smokers	31 (RR = 7)
COC users and hypertension	44 (RR = 10)

COC, combined oral contraceptive; RR, relative risk

Table 4.11 Absolute risk of non-fatal VTE in second- and third-generation pill users (per 100 000 women per annum)

Non-users	5
Second-generation COC users	15
Third-generation COC users	25
Pregnancy	60

VTE, venous thromboembolism; COC, combined oral contraceptive

the Factor V Leiden mutation, has been shown to lead to an eight-fold increase in VTE risk in non-users of COCs and a 35-fold increase in risk in association with COCs. Factor V Leiden was only discovered in the 1990s, and it is likely that there are other, as yet unrecognized inherited thrombophilic factors that will increase the risk of VTE. It therefore may be prudent simply to recommend one of the many excellent alternative forms of estrogen-free contraception to patients with a relevant personal or family history of VTE, and/or positive thrombophilia screens. Finally, it should also be remembered that the risk of fatal VTE in COC users is exceedingly low, around 1–10 per million women per year for COC users. The risk of VTE in COC users is not associated with smoking, hypertension or small varicose veins. The case fatality rate of VTE is 1–2%.

Breast cancer The risk of breast cancer is strongly associated with increasing age and is rare under the age of 40 years. Women taking COCs have a slightly higher risk of having breast cancer diagnosed than age-matched

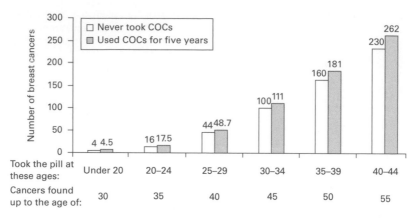

Figure 4.6 Estimated cumulative number of breast cancers per 10 000 women diagnosed in five years of use and up to 10 years after stopping combined oral contraceptives (COCs), compared with numbers of breast cancers diagnosed in 10 000 women who had never used COCs. Reproduced with permission from Schering Health Care Ltd., UK

controls: the relative risk is 1.24 (confidence interval 1.15–1.33). The estimated excess number of cancers diagnosed in the period between starting the pill and 10 years after stopping is also age-dependent and has been estimated at 0.5, 1.5 and 4.7 per 10 000 women aged 16–19, 20–24 and 25–29, respectively (Figure 4.6). Ten years after stopping the pill the excess risk of breast cancer disappears and the rate returns to the background rate. Breast cancers diagnosed in women who have taken the pill are more likely to be localized to the breast than in women who have not. It appears that women starting COCs before the age of 20 years are at higher risk than those who start them at a later stage. The risk attributable to COCs seems smallest among recent users aged 35–44 years. A higher dose (> 35 μg EE) seems to impart higher risk. The association between COCs and breast cancer is not thought to be causative. It is thought that COCs may act as growth promoters of cancers that have already arisen, or there may be earlier detection of the cancers or both.

Effective use of COCs is achieved by providing careful, accurate instructions to patients at the time of the first prescription, backed up by written information, regular revision of 'pill rules' and easy access to advice.

Cervical cancer A weak, non-causative association between COC use and cervical cancer has been demonstrated in some studies. The relative risk is 1:1 for less than 5 years of use, rising to 2.5–4.0 with more than 10 years of use. The reasons for this association are unclear. It is not known if the risk disappears if COC use is discontinued, in a way similar to breast cancer. Cervical smears should therefore be offered and carried out in accordance with local protocols.

Key examination

The only essentials for examination prior to prescribing the COC pill are blood pressure, weight and height (in order to calculate the BMI). COCs would not normally be prescribed when there is a pre-existing blood pressure equal to or greater than 140/90; a BMI of greater than 30 would be regarded as a relative contraindication, while one of 39 or over is generally considered to be an absolute contraindication. There are no data to support routine breast examination before pill prescription, nor is it necessary or desirable to carry out a vaginal examination or cervical smear before COCs are prescribed, unless indicated by appropriate factors in the history, e.g., irregular vaginal bleeding.

*Practical prescribing points
and key information for the patient*

The usual time to start taking the pill is the first day of normal bleeding of the menstrual period. When this is done, no additional contraceptive precautions are required at all. The pill can also be started any time up to day 5 of the menstrual cycle, but additional precautions, usually the use of condoms, are advised for seven days thereafter. Patients should be told to take their pill at the same time each day, ideally choosing a time at which they are most likely to remember it. If the pill is forgotten at this time, it may be taken at any time up to 12 h later without any loss of contraceptive protection. If the missed pill is forgotten for longer than 12 h, the 'missed pill' rules apply, as follows:

(1) Take the most recently forgotten pill now. Discard any earlier missed pills. Use an alternative method of contraception if intercourse occurs during the next seven days.

(2) In addition, if there are fewer than seven pills left in the pack, start the next pack without the usual break of a week between packs.

(3) And if there are seven or more pills left in the pack, when the pack is finished leave the usual seven-day break before starting the next pack.

The missed pill rules also need to be known and followed in the case of intercurrent antibiotic use, vomiting and severe diarrhea, all of which may lead to poor pill absorption and consequent lack of effect. There are anecdotal reports of pregnancies occurring after use of broad-spectrum antibiotics, such as ampicillin, tetracycline and cephalosporins. There is some evidence that the enterohepatic circulation is altered and levels of estrogen are lowered by these antibiotics which therefore reduce efficacy of the pill. Patients should be advised to follow missed pill rules whilst taking these antibiotics and for a week after

discontinuing. In the case of long-term antibiotic use, for instance in the treatment of acne, extra precautions are only required for the first fortnight after introduction of the antibiotic.

It is always a good idea to warn patients that they may experience adverse events in the first few cycles of pill taking. These episodes are usually mild and rarely persist beyond six months, but if they do, they may be alleviated by changes in the pill formulation. The reported incidence of some adverse events beyond six months is as follows: breakthrough bleeding 4–8%, breast discomfort 1–3%, nausea 1–2% and acne 1–2%; amenorrhea occurs in 0.5–1.5% of users. Patients should be advised not to stop their pills if one withdrawal bleed is missed but to seek medical advice before restarting the pill if two successive bleeds are missed. Patients also need to be advised under what circumstances they should stop pill taking immediately, use alternative contraceptive measures and take urgent medical advice. They should be advised of the symptoms that might suggest an acute cardiovascular event, such as myocardial infarction, stroke, severe migraine, pulmonary embolism or deep vein thrombosis. The other situations that may require medical advice include development of jaundice, newly diagnosed high blood pressure and elective surgery. With the latter, COCs should be discontinued four weeks beforehand if a period of immobilization is anticipated. Alternative contraception should be provided and COC use should not be restarted until at least four weeks after full mobilization.

*Follow-up of patients on combined
oral contraceptives*

New patients should be seen after three months, and subsequent visits can be at six-monthly intervals provided there are no problems. Very young patients may benefit from being seen more frequently for the first few months of pill taking. The essentials of examination at each follow-up visit are as at first prescription, i.e., measurement of blood pressure and weight. In addition, enquiry should be made about the menstrual cycle, and any unusual symptoms, such as chest or leg pain and migraine; a regular enquiry about smoking habits and family history is also advisable and advice given where necessary.

The combined contraceptive patch

A new development in combined hormonal contraception has been the development of the contraceptive patch. This is a thin, 20 cm² matrix patch that has three layers: an outer protective layer of polyester, a medicated adhesive middle layer and a clear protective layer that is removed before application. The patch delivers 20 µg of EE and 150 µg of norgestrelomine (active metabolite of norgestimate) into the systemic circulation within 24 h. The patch is changed weekly for 3 weeks followed by a patch-free week, thus forming a 28-day cycle. The patch can be applied on the upper arms, torso (excluding breasts), lower abdomen and buttocks, provided the skin is clean, dry and free of skin disorders. Each new patch should be applied away from the site of the old patch. Users can maintain their usual activities while wearing the patch, including swimming and bathing, but should not apply creams or cosmetics on or around the patch. The patch works similarly to the pill, suppression of ovulation being the main mechanism of action. In clinical studies, the user failure and method failure rates of the contraceptive patch were 1.24 and 0.99 per 100 women per year, respectively. The cycle control was good, with 3% and 1% of women experiencing breakthrough bleeding or spotting, respectively, by the end of the third cycle. These rates are very similar to those seen with the contraceptive pill. Compliance with the patch in a study setting was better than with the pill, with 89% of patients wearing the patch and 80% on COCs reporting perfect compliance. Five percent of all patches (1 in 20) had to be replaced because of partial or complete detachment. Side-effects experienced with the patch and COCs are virtually the same, apart from breast discomfort and dysmenorrhea, which is more common with the patch. Skin reactions severe enough to necessitate abandoning the method occur in 2–3% of women in clinical trials. The overall dropout rate with the patch is 25–28% which is similar to the dropout rate experienced with COCs (30%). In a year-long study of 770 women, the patch did not lead to any meaningful changes in vital signs, general and gynecologic examination patterns or laboratory parameters.

In summary, the patch is an effective method of contraception that may be useful in cases of gastrointestinal side-effects of the pill or where compliance is an issue. Clinical experience with the patch is limited and does not allow us to make any broader recommendations.

Intrauterine methods of contraception

Some of the most important advances in contraception in the past 20 years have been in intrauterine methods. Although they have the same origin, the intrauterine methods of today are more effective and have fewer side-effects as compared to the devices in use in the 1960s and 1970s. Intrauterine methods of contraception can be divided into three main types: IUDs, the intrauterine implant (IUI) and the intrauterine system (IUS) (see Table 4.12); the latter is dealt with in a separate section. To minimize the use of abbreviations, we shall sometimes use the term 'coil' instead of intrauterine contraceptive device. Examples of intrauterine devices are shown in Figure 4.7.

Worldwide, IUDs are the second most commonly used method after sterilization, although only about 4% of British women aged 15–44 choose this method, while in most other European countries rates of up to 19% are seen.

Intrauterine methods of contraception are not only highly effective but also safe, have high continuation rates, are fully and rapidly reversible, are simple to use and require no action at the time of coitus. Although some appear expensive, when considering the

Table 4.12 Intrauterine methods of contraception

Type	Devices†	Active constituent
IUD	Multiload 250 Short, Multiload 250, *Multiload 375*, Nova T 200, *Nova T 380*, T-Safe Cu 380A*	Copper
IUI	*GyneFix*	Copper
IUS	*Mirena*	Levonorgestrel

†The authors' preferred devices are in italics; *discontinued in the UK; IUD, intrauterine device; IUI, intrauterine implant; IUS, intrauterine system

overall cost for the duration of action, they are all cost-effective. Appropriately trained health care professionals should fit all intrauterine methods. The traditional IUD has a plastic T-shaped frame with a variable amount of copper in the form of wire and/or sleeves mounted on it. The plastic frame is held responsible for the menstrual disturbances associated with this contraceptive method. A recent development has been the introduction of the frameless intrauterine device GyneFix. It consists of six copper sleeves with a total surface area of 330 mm^2 threaded on polypropylene suture material. The proximal end of the thread has a knot which is buried in the fundal myometrium with an inserter for anchoring the device. The manufacturer claims that GyneFix is as effective as the best T-shaped devices, but associated with less bleeding, pain or expulsion.

Mechanism of action

Copper-containing devices The presence of copper reduces sperm motility, fertilization, and ovum development. In addition, should fertilization occur, which is rare, there is a sterile inflammatory response in the endometrium that prevents implantation. This latter mechanism is the primary effect when used for emergency contraception.

Levonorgestrel-containing devices The presence of the progestogen levonorgestrel within the uterine cavity leads to a profound suppression of the endometrium (preventing implantation),

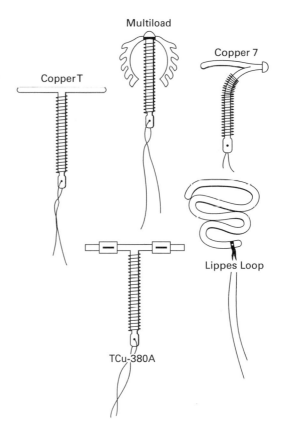

Figure 4.7 Examples of intrauterine devices. Reproduced with permission from Kleinman RL, ed. *Family Planning Handbook for Doctors*. London: International Planned Parenthood Federation, 1988:106

thickening of cervical mucus (preventing sperm migration) and a reduction in tubal motility. The plastic frame induces a foreign-body reaction.

Efficacy

The efficacy of copper-containing devices is directly related to the copper content; there is also a reduction in the rate of ectopic pregnancy in users of modern IUDs (see Table 4.13).

Copper IUDs used for emergency contraception have a failure rate in the order of 0.1 per 1000 women treated per cycle, which is superior to both hormonal methods of emergency contraception and where efficacy is important in the method of choice. The Mirena IUS is not effective as an emergency contraceptive.

Assessing suitability for intrauterine methods of contraception

Intrauterine methods of contraception are suitable for most women requesting long-term effective contraception, including many nulliparous women. There are few absolute contraindications to their use: these and the relative contraindications are listed in Tables 4.14 and 4.15.

Key history and examination

Intrauterine contraception is suitable for many women requesting contraception. The history should be taken bearing in mind the absolute and relative contraindications and should include the following.

Assessment of risk for sexually transmitted infections Risk factors for STIs include age under 25, more than one partner in the previous year, a relationship of less than previous six months' duration and, because of the possibility of treatment failure or reinfection, a recent STI. If the woman suspects or is aware that her partner is unfaithful, this also should be managed as a situation where there is an increased risk of infection. Tests for STIs may be indicated.

Assessment of menstrual problems Menorrhagia, dysmenorrhea, intermenstrual bleeding or postcoital bleeding should be investigated appropriately before insertion of an intrauterine contraceptive device.

Examination A full gynecologic and abdominal examination is carried out prior to fitting an IUD.

Complications and side-effects of using intrauterine devices

Intrauterine methods of contraception are very safe, the main risks being divided into early (i.e. at the time of fitting) and late morbidity. Mortality attributed to IUD use is very rare, 1.6 per million insertions. All the complications listed here should be discussed with the woman prior to insertion of an IUD.

Pain Most women having an IUD fitted will experience some pain or discomfort, especially when the Allis forceps is applied to the cervix, when the uterine sound is passed, and the device is inserted. Mefenamic acid 500 mg taken 30 min before fitting offers some reduction in pain. Occasionally intra-cervical local anesthesia is required. Vagal inhibition, which may rarely lead to circulatory collapse, occasionally occurs even without pain.

Uterine perforation This complication occurs in about 1 in 1000 insertions. It occurs at the time of insertion, may not be associated with pain and may go unnoticed. Perforation may be partial or complete. If not recognized at the time of insertion, the diagnosis is usually made when, at routine follow-up, the absence of threads is noted (see Missing threads, page 59).

Expulsion The rate of expulsion has been quoted at 3–15 per 100 women during the first year of use. Rates of expulsion decrease with increased age in women. Expulsion is more likely in the presence of a congenital uterine abnormality. Women should be instructed to try and feel for the threads after each period, especially during the first year of use.

Pregnancy The risk of pregnancy is greatest in the first year of use and varies according to

Table 4.13 Efficacy of intrauterine contraceptives at 2 years (various sources)

Devices	Pregnancies per 100 woman-years	Licensed duration of use (years)	Recommended maximum duration of use (years)
200 mm² copper			
Copper 7[†]	2.8	NA	NA
Nova T 200/NovaGard[†]	3.0	5	3
220 to 300 mm² copper			
Multiload 250	0.9	3	3
Copper T 220[†]	0.9	NA	NA
Flexi-T 300	1.8	5	
330 to 380 mm² copper			
GyneFix*	< 0.5	5	5
Multiload 375*	0.6	5	5
T-Safe Cu 380A*	0.3	10	12
Nova T 380*	1.6	5	5
Levonorgestrel 20 µg/24 h			
Mirena*	< 0.3	5	5

*Device recommended for routine use; [†]discontinued in the UK; NA, not available

Table 4.14 Absolute contraindications to intrauterine contraception

Pregnancy
Unexplained genital tract bleeding
Cervical or endometrial cancer
Current benign or malignant gestational
   trophoblastic disease
Cervicitis due to chlamydia or gonorrhea and
   cervicitis where these infections have not been
   excluded
Pelvic inflammatory disease current or within the
   previous 3 months
Pelvic tuberculosis
Distortion of the uterine cavity, for example by fibroids
   or congenital malformation*
Cavity length less than 5.5 cm*
Copper allergy[†]
Wilson's disease[†]

*Not necessarily a contraindication to the GyneFix intrauterine implant; [†]not a contraindication to use of the Mirena intrauterine system

Table 4.15 Relative contraindications to intrauterine contraception

At risk of sexually transmitted infections
AIDS or HIV-positive
Valvular heart disease and septal defects
   (See current British National Formulary for latest
   advice on antibiotic prophylaxis for women at
   risk of endocarditis.)
Nulliparous (small increased risk of expulsion)

*The following are relative contraindications to copper devices:**

Menorrhagia
Severe dysmenorrhea
Previous ectopic pregnancy[†]

*Mirena has a beneficial effect on these conditions; [†]not Gyne T 380 S, which is protective

the device. The most effective device is the Mirena IUS. Failure may also occur in the event of unrecognized perforation or expulsion. Self-checking of the threads by the patient can reduce the chance of failures due to these latter causes. If pregnancy occurs, it is advised that the device be removed if the threads are visible. This carries with it a risk of miscarriage, but this is not as great as the risk and consequences of septic abortion if the device remains *in utero*. Failure to remove the device is not an indication for termination of pregnancy. No teratogenic effects of IUS have been reported.

Ectopic pregnancy The IUS is protective against ectopic pregnancy and has a very low rate associated with its use. The risk of ectopic pregnancy in users of copper devices varies between devices. The lowest ectopic pregnancy rates are in those devices with more than 350 mm² copper. IUDs have a greater protective effect on intrauterine pregnancy than extrauterine pregnancy – which explains why the rate of ectopic to intrauterine pregnancies in IUD users is greater (one in 25) than in non-users of ICCDs (one in 100–200). Given these figures, should pregnancy occur in an IUD user, it is important to exclude ectopic in the first instance. However, IUDs do not cause ectopic pregnancies, and the risk of having an ectopic pregnancy is reduced with some devices such as the Gyne T 380. Mirena and the Gyne T 380 are therefore the devices of choice in women with a history of a previous ectopic pregnancy.

Actinomyces-like organisms Actinomyces is an anerobic, Gram-positive micro-organism, which is normally commensal in the mouth and the gut. The micro-organism is present in the genital tract only in the presence of an IUD. It is often found on routine cervical screening and its prevalence has been quoted between 1% and 20%, depending on the duration of use of the IUD. The presence of actinomyces-like organisms on smear does not mean that the patient has pelvic actinomycosis, but while it is thought that there may be a small increased risk, the absolute risk is negligible. Pelvic actinomycosis is very rare and the discovery of actinomyces in an asymptomatic woman does not mandate removal of the IUD. If the woman understands that she may be at a slightly higher risk of pelvic actinomycosis and prefers to be monitored for symptoms and signs once the situation has been explained to her, then the IUD can be left *in situ*. If the woman is anxious about the possibility of infection then the device should be removed or changed.

Effect on the menstrual cycle With the exception of the first few weeks after insertion,

irregular or intermenstrual bleeding is uncommon with copper devices. If abnormal bleeding does occur, the presence of displacement, partial expulsion or infection should be considered. A more usual effect is to increase the duration of menstruation and/or the menstrual loss. In some women with previously painless cycles, insertion of an IUD may lead to dysmenorrhea. The effect is not predictable and appears to be greater with ordinary IUDs than with the frameless IUI. Usual medical treatments for menorrhagia and dysmenorrhea that start after IUD insertion can be tried but these are of limited benefit in the presence of an IUD. Between 5 and 20% of IUD users will have the device removed because of problematic bleeding or pain.

Pelvic infection and intrauterine contraception

The risks of pelvic infection after insertion of an intrauterine device, system or implant are very low at approximately one case per 150–200 insertions and are only increased above the background risk in the three weeks after insertion. In fact, the risk directly attributable to the procedure may be even less. The presence of STIs increases the risk of developing PID after insertion. The Mirena actually reduces the risk of developing PID, and the risk associated with the GyneFix has not been fully evaluated but appears to be lower than that associated with conventional coils. The importance of PID is two-fold. Firstly, every episode of PID carries with it a significant risk of subsequent subfertility or ectopic pregnancy secondary to tubal damage. Secondly, PID is an unpleasant condition that causes pain and may cause a systemic illness. Because of the association with STIs, many cases of PID post insertion are potentially preventable. Some doctors advise screening all women for chlamydia prior to insertion if there is a prevalence of chlamydia of 3% or greater in the local population. However, this is not the practice of the authors as it can delay fitting and is not appropriate for all women.

It is important that all women having an IUD fitted are informed beforehand of the risks of PID and helped to put their own individual risk into perspective, with testing for STIs if appropriate.

Management of pelvic inflammatory disease after insertion of an intrauterine device

PID is a clinical diagnosis (see Appendix II for details of diagnosis, investigation and management). If the woman with PID wishes to continue to use the IUD as her method of contraception, it should not be removed. Treatment should be commenced and the patient reassessed after 48–72 h. At this time there will be improvement in most women; however, if this is not the case, the diagnosis should be reconsidered and if no other cause of PID is found, the IUD should then probably be removed to facilitate a cure.

Missing threads

If the patient reports that she cannot feel the threads or if the threads are not seen during examination, there are four possibilities: (1) the threads are present, have curled up and are lying in the cervical canal or the uterine cavity; (2) pregnancy; (3) expulsion; or (4) perforation. Pregnancy can be confirmed or excluded either by the history, a clinical examination and/or a pregnancy test. Until the position of the IUD is confirmed, the woman should be advised to use an alternative method of contraception. Sometimes the threads can be identified just in the os; unless the IUD is to be removed it is not advised to try to bring the threads down as this may dislodge the IUD. If the woman is not pregnant and the threads cannot be found, a pelvic ultrasound scan should be performed. The result will show the coil present either inside the uterus or outside, in the pelvis, or absent. If the coil is in the uterus and not displaced, all that is needed are six-monthly ultrasound scans to reassure the patient that the device is still in the uterus. The woman should report any unusual bleeding or pain. If the coil is outside the uterus in the pelvis, it needs to be removed surgically, usually laparoscopically, but occasionally laparotomy is required. If the coil is absent, a plain abdominal X-ray should be performed to ensure it is not intra-abdominal; if not, expulsion is assumed and a new coil may be fitted or a different method of contraception advised.

Timing of insertion

The usual time to insert a copper coil is just post-menstrual or during the menses. The latter is associated with a very slightly higher expulsion rate. However, it can be inserted at any time of the cycle, provided there is no risk that a pregnancy has already implanted (see Intrauterine emergency contraception, page 73).

Removal of intrauterine devices

To avoid pregnancy, IUDs are best removed during menses and when another method of contraception has been initiated. They should not be removed mid-cycle if intercourse has taken place in the previous seven days because of a theoretical risk of pregnancy.

Progestogen-only contraception

During the last 10 years, there has been a great expansion in the range of progestogen-only methods available. At the time of writing, there are short term, long-term and emergency methods of progestogen-only contraception. In some cases the efficacy of the long-term method equals or exceeds that of sterilization. All progestogen-only methods have minimal metabolic effects that are not significant clinically, meaning that they can be used safely in older women and those who have contraindications to estrogen-containing contraceptives. They often require minimal user compliance and little doctor or nurse involvement after the initial consultation. The main side effect common to all progestogen-only methods is unpredictable bleeding: this will be discussed in more detail under individual methods.

Progestogen-only pill

Mode of action   Second- and third-generation progestogen-only pills (POPs) are now available on the market. The second-generation POPs contain the progestogens norgestrel, levonorgestrel, norethisterone or ethynodiol and the third-generation POPs contain desogestrel.

The principal effect of second-generation POPs is on the cervical mucus, causing increased viscosity and sperm impenetrability. This effect is exquisitely sensitive to the serum progestogen concentration and therefore meticulous, regular pill taking is required to ensure consistent serum levels. It is generally accepted that the effect on cervical mucus wears off 27 h after taking a pill. To be effective, at least two pills must have been taken correctly. Other effects of second-generation POPs are on the endometrium in which normal thickening and maturation do not occur, leading to failure of implantation if fertilization does occur, decreased fallopian tube motility, and, in approximately 15% of women, suppression of ovulation.

All of the above mentioned mechanisms of action apply to the third-generation POPs as well; however, for these agents the rate of ovulation suppression is considerably higher, i.e., over 95%.

Efficacy and drug interactions   Failure rates for second-generation POPs are age-related and range from < 1 per 100 woman-years in women over 35 years, up to 4–5 per 100 woman-years in those under 25 years. This difference is likely to be caused by a combination of factors, including falling fertility and higher pill-taking reliability in older women. Users can be advised that there are no interactions with commonly used antibiotics. For POPs containing desogestrel, the overall failure rate is estimated at 0.4/100 woman-years.

Some studies suggest that there may be a weight-related increase in failure rates of hormonal methods, such as POPs and COCs. As a result, some clinicians advise the use of two tablets daily in women weighing over 70 kg. This matter is hotly debated, with the Summary of Product Characteristics advising against the practice. An analysis of the Oxford Family Planning Association database did not find a correlation between weight and failure rate either.

Key history, indications and contraindications
The following should be considered:

(1)   All women requesting hormonal contraception should have a medical and family history taken as detailed in the section on combined oral contraception.

(2)   There are in practice no absolute contraindications to POPs, although pregnancy should be excluded before commencing treatment and undiagnosed vaginal bleeding should always be investigated appropriately before commencing any hormonal method of contraception.

(3)   A history of ectopic pregnancy is a relative contraindication only because ovulation is not reliably suppressed and tubal motility is reduced. Thus, if fertilization does occur there is an increased risk of ectopic implantation; the ectopic rate is nevertheless lower than in women not using contraception.

(4)   The POP is particularly suitable for women in the following categories:

(a)   Lactating women;

(b)   Personal or immediate family history of VTE;

(c)   Women over 35 years with risk factors for combined oral contraception, e.g., smokers, those with cardiovascular risk factors such as diabetes or hypertension;

(d)   Migraine sufferers who experience aura or severe migraine headaches;

(e)   Overweight individuals;

(f)   As a matter of choice for any woman who is a reliable pill taker.

Examination, choice of pill and prescribing information Provided that the history is normal, all that need be determined at an examination are blood pressure and weight. Blood pressure is not generally influenced in any way by POPs but where there is pre-existing hypertension, careful monitoring is indicated. The more androgenic levonorgestrel (as found in Microval/Neogest) may be more likely to increase blood pressure than norethisterone (as found in Micronor/Noriday).

The actual choice of POP for any individual patient is fairly arbitrary and is made on an empirical basis. Any of the brands listed in Table 4.16 may be used as first choice, with the opportunity to switch to an alternative progestogen if the bleeding pattern or any other side-effects are unacceptable. Ethynodiol diacetate (the progestogen in Femulen) is a pro-drug, metabolized to norethisterone, and has no particular advantages.

Key prescribing points are as follows:

(1) Pill-taking should be commenced on day 1 of menses; and when this happens, no additional precautions are needed.

(2) Pills are taken continuously, without any break at any time in the cycle.

(3) Pills should be taken regularly within three hours of the same time each day. The actual time of day is not crucial. The most important factor is the likelihood of the woman remembering the chosen time.

(4) If a pill is taken more than 3 h later than the regular time, the effectiveness of contraceptive cover will be reduced. Current advice is to take the forgotten pill as soon as possible, to continue taking pills at the regular time and to use extra contraceptive precautions for seven days.

(5) Menstrual irregularity may occur and is unpredictable, ranging from amenorrhea, through infrequent bleeding, fairly normal regular cycles to frequent and/or heavy bleeding. Approximately 50% of women will have a fairly normal cycle and only a small number have bleeding problems.

Table 4.16 Progestogen-only pills

Proprietary name	Progestogen	Dose (µg)
Microval	Levonorgestrel	30
Norgeston	Levonorgestrel	30
Neogest	Norgestrel	75
Micronor	Norethisterone	350
Noriday	Norethisterone	350
Femulen	Ethynodiol diacetate	500
Cerazette	Desogestrel	75

(6) Minor side-effects include slight breast tenderness at the onset of pill-taking and other progestogenic effects such as acne, headaches and bloating.

(7) Functional ovarian cysts are more common in POP users than in those not using this hormonal method. Whilst most functional ovarian cysts are asymptomatic and spontaneously resolve, they may present with abdominal pain.

(8) Follow-up of POP users includes regular weighing, annual blood pressure taking provided it remains normal, and assessment of menstrual pattern.

(9) POP use can be started 2–3 weeks after delivery.

Injectable contraception

Injectable progestogen-only contraception is now widely used. There are two such preparations available in the UK – one containing medroxyprogesterone acetate (Depo-Provera) and the other norethisterone enanthate (Noristerat; see Table 4.17). There are no combined injectable estrogen/progestogen contraceptives licensed in the UK. Originally both available progestogen-only injectable contraceptives were licensed only for short-term use, i.e., for women whose partners had undergone vasectomy and were awaiting confirmation of sterility, for women awaiting sterilization or following rubella immunization. A general licence for Depo-Provera was granted in the UK in 1995.

Table 4.17 Injectable progestogen-only contraceptives

Product name	Progestogen	Dose (µg)	Injection interval
Depo-Provera	Medroxyprogesterone acetate	150	Every 12 weeks (± 5 days)
Noristerat	Norethisterone enanthate	200	Every 8 weeks (± 5 days)

Norethisterone enanthate is still licensed for short-term use after vasectomy but is used more widely for women who want an injectable method but who have experienced side-effects with medroxyprogesterone acetate.

Mode of action and efficacy Injectable progestogens work primarily on the hypothalamic–pituitary–ovarian axis to suppress gonadotropin production and thus prevent ovarian follicular development and ovulation; they also share with other progestogen-only methods effects on the endometrium (atrophy), fallopian tubes (reduced motility) and cervical mucus (thickening). They have a very high efficacy, with failure rates between < 0.01 and 1.5 per 100 woman-years, which is at least comparable to that of sterilization and, because ovulation is inhibited, there is no relative increase in ectopic rates.

Key history, indications and contraindications These are essentially the same as for POPs. Caution should be used before recommending injectables for women with a history of severe postnatal or endogenous depression as some authorities consider that depression may recur on injectable preparations; this has not been the authors' experience. They should not be used for any woman planning a pregnancy in the near future, due to possible delay in return of fertility (see below); neither are they suitable for women not prepared to tolerate menstrual irregularity or amenorrhea. However, injectables may be particularly suitable for the following groups of women:

(1) Young women requiring long-term, reliable contraception, particularly where difficulties exist with regard to remembering to take pills;

(2) Women with homozygous (SS) and SC sickle cell disease, in whom the hematologic profile is improved and the frequency of sickle cell crises is reduced by Depo-Provera;

(3) Women who cannot take estrogen-containing contraception, e.g., those with a history of VTE or coagulation risk due to conditions such as systemic lupus erythematosus or known thrombophilia;

(4) Women who develop hypertension on the combined oral contraceptive;

(5) Postnatally, as injectables do not diminish, and may even increase, milk production (but see below, under prescribing details).

Examination, choice of injectable and prescribing information Blood pressure and weight as for POPs; breast and pelvic examination and cervical smear only if appropriate or clinically indicated.

The usual first-choice injectable is Depo-Provera; however, Noristerat does have certain advantages over Depo-Provera. In particular, it is thought to cause less weight gain (although hard evidence is lacking), a greater likelihood of regular cycles and, lastly, the return of regular menstruation following cessation of treatment is usually more rapid. Against these advantages is the drawback of an oily preparation which is more difficult and painful to inject and has to be repeated every eight weeks as compared to every 12 weeks.

Key prescribing points are as follows:

(1) The first injection should be given on day 1 of menses, in which case no additional precautions are needed; if started

between day 2 and day 5 extra precautions should be used for 7 days.

(2) Postpartum, the first injection should ideally be given after six weeks. An immediate postpartum injection may lead to unacceptably prolonged bleeding, although in individual cases it may be appropriate to give it at 21 days postpartum.

(3) Following first-trimester termination the injection can be given immediately.

(4) Subsequent injections should be given at the recommended intervals (see Table 4.17).

Patients should be advised of the following:

(1) Menstrual change is very common; amenorrhea is the commonest pattern, but frequent and/or prolonged bleeding may occur, particularly during the first three to six months (for management, see below). Amenorrhea occurs in 30, 55 and 68% of women after 3, 12 and 24 months of use, respectively. Prolonged heavy bleeding requiring treatment is noted in 0.5–4 per 100 woman-years.

(2) Regular use of Depo-Provera may lead to less premenstrual tension, less dysmenorrhea and less anemia.

(3) Weight gain, probably due to appetite stimulation, and a reduction in the volume of blood loss, are the commonest reasons for discontinuation of the method. The weight gain is in the region of 2–3 kg after 1–2 years of use, rising to 6–7 kg after 4–6 years of use.

(4) After the last injection, there may be a delay in the return of normal menstrual cycles and possibly fertility, very rarely up to 18 months; there is no effect on long-term fertility.

Amenorrhea owing to Depo-Provera use may also be associated in the long term with hypo-estrogenism, which carries the theoretical risk of decreased bone mineral density (and consequent fracture risk) and an increased risk of ischemic heart disease. While some studies have demonstrated a reduction in bone density in women using Depo-Provera, this has not been borne out in other studies. No increase in ischemic heart disease has been seen in studies specifically looking at this.

Drug interactions   There is no good evidence that liver enzyme-inducing drugs, including certain anti-epileptic therapies such as carbamazepine, griseofulvin and rifampicin, lead to a reduced efficacy of Depo-Provera. Current medical practice, however, is to err on the side of caution and advise injections at reduced intervals, i.e. every 10 weeks. This reduction in interval times applies to rifampicin, even if only a single dose is given, as hepatic enzymes can be induced for up to four weeks. Extra contraceptive precautions should be also be used for that period of time.

Management of prolonged bleeding on Depo-Provera
In cases where there is prolonged bleeding after a Depo-Provera injection, it is necessary to exclude other causes of bleeding, such as pregnancy and infection. Provided estrogen is not contraindicated, bleeding can usually be controlled by additional estrogen therapy. This is most conveniently done by taking one packet of any low-dose COC pill. This will frequently be effective and the next injection can then be given at the normal time; if the next injection is due in less than four weeks, it can be given early and the patient reassured that the bleeding will almost invariably settle down after this next injection.

Implants

One progestogen-only implant is now available in the UK, namely Implanon. This is a single rod system, 4 cm long and 2 mm wide (Figure 4.8). It contains a core of 68 mg etonogestrel enclosed in an ethylenevinylacetate (EVA) membrane which is non-biodegradable. It is designed for the slow, controlled release of

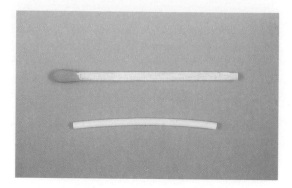

Figure 4.8 Size of Implanon subdermal implant in relation to a matchstick. Reproduced with permission from Organon, UK

etonogestrel over a period of three years. Pre-launch studies demonstrated Implanon to be a highly effective contraceptive with no pregnancies occurring in over 90 000 cycles of use. The Pearl index with normal use is therefore likely to be very low and approaching zero. A progesterone-only implant called Norplant, which was launched in 1993, was removed from the UK market by the manufacturer for commercial reasons in 1999, but it is still available through some suppliers who import it.

Mode of action The principal mode of action of Implanon is inhibition of ovulation; this occurs via suppression of LH secretion from the pituitary gland. In one study, complete suppression of ovulation occurred during the first two years of Implanon use, while in the last (third) year, ovulation was suppressed in more than 95% of users. Despite the suppression of ovulation, ovarian activity continues as FSH levels are not significantly affected, with the result that normal estradiol levels are maintained. There are also – in common with all progestogen-only methods – effects on cervical mucus with increased viscosity leading to reduced sperm penetration and a reduction in the thickness of the endometrium, both of which contribute to contraceptive efficacy.

Key history, examination and contraindications Implanon should be considered for women wanting long-term, highly effective but reversible contraception. As it invariably causes alteration in the menstrual pattern, it is not suitable for women not prepared to tolerate this. It is likely to prove popular with young women who do not wish to become pregnant for some years and want a method that requires minimal patient or health professional involvement. It should not be used if pre-existing pregnancy is suspected, nor in the presence of undiagnosed vaginal bleeding or hormone-dependent tumors. It is contraindicated in active venous thromboembolic disorders but can be given to women with a history of VTE who wish to use hormonal contraception.

Drug interactions There may be interactions with potent enzyme inducers such as rifampicin, griseofulvin, phenytoin and carbamazepine; nospecific interaction studies have been performed on Implanon, and advice on its use is based on extrapolation from studies of other progestogen-only methods. If enzyme inducers are concurrently prescribed then an alternative method of contraception is advisable. If only short-term use of enzyme inducers is planned, then barrier method(s) should additionally be used when the enzyme inducer is prescribed.

Timing of Implanon injections The following should be considered:

(1) In women previously using barrier methods of contraception or no method at all, the injection should be given in the first five days of the cycle. If injected later than day 2 of the cycle, extra contraceptive precautions should be used for the first seven days.

(2) In women transferring from combined oral contraception, the injection should be given during the pill-free week, while in women transferring from another progestogen-only method, it can be injected at any time, provided the patient and operator are confident that an ongoing pregnancy is not present. In the case of transfer from the POP, extra

precautions should be used for the following seven days.

(3) In IUD users, Implanon can be injected at any time while the IUD is in place, the IUD device then being removed with the next menstrual period.

(4) Following pregnancy, Implanon can be injected immediately after first-trimester termination, whilst after later terminations and full-term deliveries it is recommended that the injection should be delayed until 21–28 days after delivery.

Insertion Following infiltration of 5 ml of local anesthetic, the implant is inserted subdermally 6–8 cm above the elbow in the inner aspect of the non-dominant arm using the preloaded applicator (Figures 4.9 and 4.10) and following the manufacturer's instructions, which should be supplemented by supervised training. The injection site should be kept covered and dry for the first 24–48 h; a pressure bandage may help to prevent any bruising.

Bleeding pattern and side-effects Consider the following:

(1) An unpredictable bleeding pattern should be expected, both between users and within the same user.

(2) Approximately 20% of women will have amenorrhea at some point during use.

(3) Approximately 25% will have infrequent bleeding at some point during use.

(4) Approximately 10% will have prolonged episodes of bleeding and spotting at some point during use.

(5) Less than 10% will have frequent bleeding or spotting (more than six bleeding episodes in a 90-day period) at some point during use.

(6) A mean weight increase of 1–2% per year has been reported. This does not differ significantly from the weight increase seen

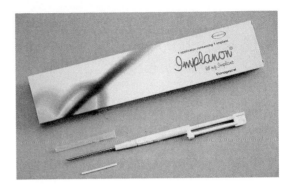

Figure 4.9 Implanon subdermal implant (with applicator). Reproduced with permission from Organon, UK

in women using non-hormonal methods of contraception over the same period.

(7) Where there is pre-existing acne, the condition generally improves with Implanon use, but in a small (approximately 10%) proportion of women it may worsen; in less than 15% of women acne may appear for the first time.

(8) Mood changes, breast tenderness, headaches and nausea occur in some Implanon users, in common with all hormonal methods.

(9) Loss of libido and hair thinning or actual hair loss have also been reported.

Removal and return of fertility Implanon is removed using a small skin incision under local anesthesia. The process may leave a small scar (2–3 mm). It is the correct and careful subdermal insertion that determines the ease of removal of the rod. Excluding the duration of the anesthetic application, the mean time needed for the insertion of Implanon is 1.1 min and for removal it is 2.6 min. Return of fertility is very rapid and this is one of the advantages of this method compared to injectable contraception; in studies, over 94% of women ovulated within three weeks of removal of the implant. Thus, an alternative method of contraception or a new implant should be used immediately, unless a pregnancy is planned.

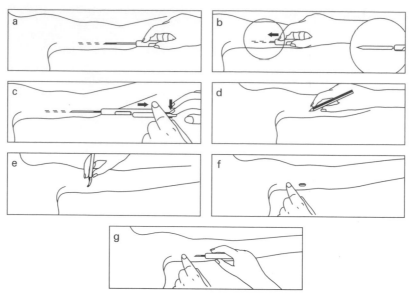

Figure 4.10 Insertion (a, b and c) and removal (d, e, f and g) of Implanon. Reproduced with permission from Organon, UK

Intrauterine progestogen-only methods

The Mirena IUS is a levonorgestrel-releasing IUD which should be included in the progestogen-only methods category rather than 'intrauterine devices', its mode of action being different from that of copper IUDs, relating rather to the progestogen content. Introduced into the UK in 1995, Mirena has rapidly become a popular method of contraception, particularly with women requiring long-term contraception or those considering sterilization.

Mirena intrauterine system – mode of action The Mirena IUS releases 20 μg levonorgestrel per 24 h into the endometrial cavity (Figure 4.11). It has several different contraceptive mechanisms including: (1) profound suppression of the endometrium with atrophy of endometrial glands and mucosal thinning; (2) thickening of cervical mucus; and (3) inhibition of sperm motility and function. The cumulative effect of these changes is to prevent fertilization from occurring, with the additional safety feature of an inactive endometrium preventing implantation should fertilization occur.

Evidence from studies looking for transient rises in human chorionic gonadotropin show that fertilization does not occur, which indicates that there is prevention rather than interruption of implantation. There is a variable effect on ovarian function with suppression of ovulation being most common during the first year of use. However, with long-term use, more than two-thirds of cycles are ovulatory. The bleeding pattern that occurs with IUS use does not relate to ovarian function but rather to the endometrial effects of the system. There is probably an additional foreign-body effect of the device itself, which may play a minor part in exerting a contraceptive effect.

Key history, indications and contraindications Many of the contraindications to IUD (see page 56) apply equally to the IUS but there are important differences. For example, a history of menorrhagia, with or without dysmenorrhea, would be a contraindication to all copper-bearing coils while it would act as a specific indication for the levonorgestrel-releasing IUS. Similarly, an intolerance of all hormonal methods would be a contraindication to the IUS while being, in general, an indication for a coil.

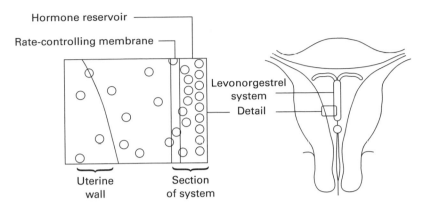

Figure 4.11 Diffusion of levonorgestrel from the intrauterine system Mirena to the endometrium. Reproduced with permission from Schering Oy, Finland

The history should be taken as though the woman was requesting hormonal contraception (bearing in mind also any specific contraindications relating to the use of intrauterine devices: see page 56). The IUS will be particularly suitable for the following:

(1) Current IUD users with heavy periods.

(2) Other patients with heavy periods (if otherwise suitable for an IUD).

(3) Patients wanting long-term contraception who:

    (a) Cannot remember to take pills regularly;

    (b) Cannot take estrogens;

    (c) Find weight gain on Depo-Provera unacceptable;

    (d) Do not want an implant;

    (e) Have a complete family, but find sterilization too final.

(4) Patients who will accept:

    (a) The possibility of irregular bleeding in the first 3 months, and rarely longer;

    (b) Amenorrhea, should it occur.

A history of ectopic pregnancy is not a contraindication to the IUS. The rates of ectopic pregnancy occurring with the IUS *in situ* are extremely low, with studies recording a rate of 0.1–0.02 per 100 woman-years in IUS users, compared to 0.2–0.6 per 100 woman-years in users of copper-releasing IUDs. The rate of ectopic pregnancy in women using no contraception is about one in 100 to one in 200, i.e., at least ten-fold higher than in IUS users. In a major study carried out by the Population Council, there were no ectopic pregnancies with the Mirena IUS during 3416 contraceptive years of exposure. The possibility of ectopic pregnancy should not be ignored, however.

Key prescribing information The IUS is associated with approximately a 40% reduction in menstrual loss, making this method particularly suitable for women suffering from menorrhagia. Initially, there is often frequent and prolonged light spotting, interspersed with light regular menstrual periods. After three to six months, as endometrial atrophy develops, the bleeding pattern usually settles to light, regular bleeds with no intermenstrual spotting; in at least 20% of women, amenorrhea develops by the twelfth month of use. The bleeding pattern that is seen is related to the endometrial suppression, with concomitant lack of estrogen responsiveness, rather than to changes in ovarian function. Estrogens and progestogens are used in various guises to manage the bleeding should it become troublesome for the patient; however, none has been shown to have a predictably beneficial effect. In the longer term, in association with the marked reduction in menstrual loss, there is a rise in hemoglobin and ferritin levels. As with all progestogen-only methods, functional ovarian cysts may occur which are usually self-limiting. If identified coincidentally on pelvic ultrasound scan they are generally managed conservatively, intervention being restricted to those which undergo complications such as torsion, hemorrhage or rupture. Other progestational side-effects such as transient breast tenderness, hirsutism, acne and mood changes may occur; they are commonest during the first three months after insertion and rarely lead to discontinuation of the method. No differences in weight gain have been seen in comparative studies of IUS and copper IUD users. There is a suggestion that pelvic infection rates may be reduced in IUS users, although this has not been confirmed in all studies. Some perimenopausal women with meno-/metrorrhagia choose the IUS with the dual aim of contraception and improved vaginal bleeding pattern. In such cases the meno-/metrorrhagia should be investigated first, so no malignancy is missed.

Efficacy and drug interactions The IUS is a highly effective contraceptive, which does not require user compliance and which, once fitted, requires little medical intervention. In a variety of studies, both comparative and non-comparative, a Pearl index of less than 0.3 has been reported, indicating that the IUS is at least as effective as female sterilization. Little is known about the effect of hepatic enzyme inducers on the efficacy of the IUS, but because its action is mainly local, some authorities believe that efficacy will be maintained and that, after appropriate counseling, the Mirena IUS can be used in women taking concurrent enzyme inducers.

Practical prescribing matters The Mirena IUS should ideally be inserted on day 1 of the menstrual cycle and then there is no need for extra contraceptive measures. It can be inserted up to day 7, but extra contraceptive precautions should then be used for seven days after insertion. If there has been no sexual intercourse in the cycle and pregnancy can definitely be excluded then the Mirena can be inserted at any time during the cycle, with additional precautions until the next period, the expected time of the next period or for three weeks if these are not definable. It is not, however, suitable for use as a post-coital contraceptive. Patients requiring emergency contraception who also wish to use the Mirena as a long-term method should be offered standard oral emergency contraception or fitted with a copper IUD, with the Mirena IUS being substituted at the time of the next menstrual period. Postpartum insertion of the IUS is recommended at 6 weeks and there is no evidence of any deleterious effect on the breastfed infant. Following first-trimester abortion, the IUS can be inserted immediately.

The method of fitting a Mirena IUS is by means of a special inserter which is claimed to be easier to use. The inserter is different from those used for IUDs and one must follow the manufacturer's instructions. As the inserter tube is wider than for the above IUDs – approximately 4.8 mm in diameter – the cervical canal may require gentle dilatation, which can be done without anesthesia, using standard Hegar dilators up to size 5. If anesthesia is required this is best provided with intracervical infiltration of local anesthetic. Some use intracervical xylocaine gel.

Follow-up is advised at four to six weeks after insertion, six months and then yearly until it is time to replace the device, which under the present license is at 5 years. It can be replaced immediately with a new IUS if desired. At each follow-up visit, enquiry should be made about the menstrual pattern, any untoward side-effects, and the patient's weight should be recorded. Patients who have become amenorrheic should have pregnancy excluded and be reassured. Return of fertility after removal of the IUS is rapid, with the majority of women re-establishing normal menstrual cycles within one month after removal, and conception rates during the following year are comparable with those seen after cessation of other contraceptive methods. There have been no reports of birth defects caused by Mirena use in cases where pregnancy continues to term with the device in place.

New developments in hormonal contraception

A monthly vaginal contraceptive ring releasing EE and etonogestrel is in an advanced stage of development. It is likely that in the future progestogen-only methods of contraception based on the newer progestogens will appear. Monthly and six-monthly injectable contraceptives are currently being developed and some (Cyclofem, Chinese, Perlutal) are already available in some countries.

STERILIZATION

Sterilization is still the most widely used method of contraception in couples over 40 years old in the UK. As long-acting and reversible methods such as the Mirena, Implanon and the newer copper IUDs are increasingly recognized as being not only highly effective but also acceptable, they are likely to challenge female sterilization as the method of choice for women who have completed their family. Another important point to note is that in many areas of the UK reversal of sterilization is not available on the National Health Service.

Any person undergoing sterilization must be willing to accept that it is permanent. The family planning provider has the responsibility to ensure that the person considering sterilization has real expectations from the procedure, with regard to permanence, failure rates (in comparison with other methods) and complications. This means that the doctor or nurse giving family planning advice must have a good understanding of all currently available long-acting methods of contraception.

Male sterilization

Vasectomy is the most effective established method of contraception currently available,

with a failure rate ranging from 1:2000 to 1:10 000 after two azoospermic samples. It is suitable for men who have completed their family and, rarely, for those who have decided not to have children. It is usually carried out under local anesthesia and has very few contraindications. Briefly, the procedure can be described in the following way: After anesthetizing the skin, the vas deferens is identified and immobilized through the scrotum. After that, the scrotum is opened. In conventional vasectomy the surgeon uses a scalpel to make two incisions in the scrotal skin, one over each vas deferens. The incisions are 1–2 cm long. The vas is brought out into the open. About a 1 cm portion of the vas is removed and both ends are ligated. The entry incisions are then closed with sutures. In a 'no-scalpel' vasectomy, the scrotum is entered bluntly with a special sharp hemostat rather than a scalpel. This creates a small puncture wound that does not need suturing. Fewer complications and less pain are reported with the 'no-scalpel' vasectomy. There has been much discussion and research into a possible link between vasectomy and prostatic cancer but such a link has now been disproved, reinforcing the safety of this important method of contraception. Reversal should be discussed before the surgery, in regard to both its availability and success rates. Reversal of sterilization defined as the presence of sperm in the ejaculate is successful in 70–92% of cases depending on the technique, the surgeon's experience, the time that has elapsed since the vasectomy and the type of vasectomy procedure. Reversal of sterilization defined as pregnancy rate is much lower, with rates between 25–80% being reported. There is also inter-surgeon variation in success rates.

Vasectomy is not immediately effective, because of the length of sperm survival. The vas distal to the vasectomy contains viable spermatozoa for weeks after the operation. Patients must be aware of this and receive advice about effective interim contraception. About 20 ejaculations are needed to clear the remaining sperm. Clearance is delayed by abstinence from ejaculation. It is usual to carry

Table 4.18 Complications of vasectomy

(1) Wound complications

    (a) pain (significant in 8%)
    (b) bleeding/hematoma (4%)
    (c) infection (2%)

(2) Failure, early/late*
(3) Post-vasectomy pain syndrome (3–8%)
(4) Possible psychologic effects/regret

*Early failure is defined as pregnancy occuring within six months after the operation or before azoospermia is docmented. Late failure is defined as pregnancy occuring after this period

Table 4.19 Complications of female sterilization

Complication	Approximate frequency
Regret	6%
Mortality	1–2 per 100 000
Damage to bowel or vascular tree	1 in 1000
Thromboembolism	Rare
Wound infection	1–2%
Ectopic pregnancy rate	10% of failures

out semen analyses at 12 and 16 weeks post vasectomy. After two consecutive negative semen analyses one month apart the vasectomy can be regarded as being successful. If the samples fail to clear, then early reanastomosis or an additional unidentified vas is present and re-operation may be required.

Men who seek a vasectomy should be advised that:

(1) Vasectomy is not castration and does not affect sexual ability or cause impotence.

(2) After vasectomy, the man continues to ejaculate because sperm contribute by only 10% to the volume of the ejaculate.

(3) Vasectomy does not cause prostatic cancer or early atherosclerosis.

The complications of a vasectomy procedure are listed in Table 4.18. Sperm granuloma is a small nodule that forms when sperm leak out of the vas deferens or the epididymis, inducing an inflammatory reaction. Post-vasectomy pain syndrome is defined as chronic pain in the testis following a vasectomy. Conservative treatment with non-steroidal anti-inflammatory medication, sitz baths or spermatic cord block may help.

Female sterilization

The convenience and efficacy of this method have made it the most commonly used single method in women over 40 who have a completed family. Recent data from the USA indicate that the failure rate of female sterilization is higher than previously thought: at around one in 200 over 10 years. Failure rates are highest in women sterilized under the age of 35 or at the time of Cesarean section, in the puerperium or at the time of termination of pregnancy. There may also be more regret in those having sterilization in association with a recent pregnancy. The risks of sterilization are small but quantifiable (see Table 4.19). Sterilization is particularly suitable for women who:

(1) Have completed their family;

(2) Find no other long-term method acceptable;

(3) Have no gynecologic condition that requires hysterectomy;

(4) Have no conditions that make the procedure dangerous (for example, obesity).

Sterilization is usually carried out under general anesthesia. It is effected by applying clips or rings to the isthmus of the fallopian tubes. Diathermy is rarely used now because of the risk of damaging intra-abdominal organs. Partial salpingectomy (modified Pomeroy technique) requires a mini-laparotomy and is particularly useful in countries where laparoscopy is not available, and it can also be done as a day case. An important risk is that of ectopic pregnancy should failure occur, and a woman who has previously been sterilized and who is pregnant should have a scan at four to five weeks' gestation to locate the pregnancy.

There is usually a delay between the decision to be sterilized and the actual operation; an effective interim contraceptive is required because some women become pregnant while waiting for the procedure to be done. In addition, a sterilization carried out in the luteal phase of the cycle carries a theoretical risk of an ectopic pregnancy if a fertilized ovum is still within the tube distal to the clip.

After laparoscopic sterilization, women can expect some abdominal discomfort and shoulder pain for up to a week. Women who have been using a method that makes menstruation lighter (such as the COC pill) or absent (such as depo-medroxyprogesterone acetate) and are opting for sterilization should be advised that their periods may appear to get heavier when that method is discontinued – and in some cases this could be unacceptable.

As with the reversal of vasectomy, the success of the reversal of female sterilization varies depending on the amount of tube damaged by the initial procedure and the surgical technique used for the original operation.

EMERGENCY CONTRACEPTION

Emergency contraception is a useful means of preventing unplanned pregnancy after unprotected sexual contact or potential contraceptive failure (see Table 4.20). Although pregnancy is unlikely before day 7 of the cycle or after day 17 of the cycle in a woman with a 28-day cycle, any request for emergency contraception should be assessed for risk based on Table 4.20 and – if indicated – emergency contraception offered.

Whilst having been demonstrated to be effective if commenced any time up to 72 h after sex, the efficacy of the hormonal methods (Levonelle-2 and Schering PC4) declines with time after intercourse. Because of this, a request for emergency contraception should – wherever possible – be dealt with at the time of the request. On-call services and accident and emergency departments are therefore important points for accessing emergency contraception. Furthermore, Lev-

Table 4.20 Indications for emergency contraception

Unprotected sex (consensual or non-consensual)

(1) Intercourse where contraceptive method was not used or used incorrectly
(2) Coitus interruptus
(3) After rape or sexual assault
(4) Ejaculation on to external genitalia

Potential contraceptive failure

(1) COCs
  (a) two or more pills missed from first seven of the pack
  (b) four or more pills missed mid-pack
  (c) potential drug interaction

(2) POPs
  (a) one or more pills missed (taken more than 3 h late)
  (b) potential drug interaction

(3) IUDs
  (a) expulsion (partial or complete)
  (b) mid-cycle removal after intercourse in previous seven days

(4) Barriers
  (a) condom split, slippage or incorrect use
  (b) diaphragm split, displacement or incorrect use

COC, combined oral contraceptive; POP, progestogen-only pill; IUD, intrauterine device

onelle-2 can be bought over the counter for emergency use. Good access to emergency IUDs is important, and all services offering hormonal methods should have access, by referral if necessary, to this method.

Efficacy of emergency contraception

The efficacy of emergency contraception can be expressed either as the chance of pregnancy after using the method, or as the ratio of observed to expected pregnancies. The latter is used in this text.

Methods of emergency contraception

There are three main methods of emergency contraception: two hormonal and one intrauterine.

Progestogen-only hormonal emergency contraceptives

Licensed in 1999, Levonelle-2 is the most recent advance in the provision of emergency contraception in the UK. It consists of two doses, each of one tablet containing 750 µg of levonorgestrel. The first dose is commenced within 72 h of intercourse and the second 12 h later. A recent randomized controlled trial involving over 4000 women showed that 1.5 mg of levonorgestrel taken as a single dose may be as effective as the usual regimen.

Efficacy Current evidence indicates that this is the more effective of the hormonal methods, with 86% of expected pregnancies prevented when started within 72 h of intercourse. As with the Schering PC4, the efficacy is higher the earlier it is started (see Table 4.21). Hepatic enzyme-inducing agents may reduce efficacy and an IUD should be considered. Efficacy may also be reduced if the patient vomits within 2 h of taking either dose.

It is improtant to remember that progestogen-only emergency contraceptives have some efficacy even beyond 72 h and up to 120 h. One estimate is 50–60%. It is a 'better than nothing' method for those women who present after 72 h, but are unable or unwilling to have an IUD fitted.

Prescribing Levonelle-2 The manufacturers advise that pregnancy, severe cardiovascular disease (arterial or venous), acute focal migraine and severe liver disease are contraindicated to the use of Levonelle-2.

Follow-up of patients It is usual to advise patients after use of emergency contraception to return in three weeks to exclude pregnancy. In practice, however, most patients do not return. It is therefore probably more important to ensure they are aware of what symptoms should lead them to seek medical advice should pregnancy occur. These include amenorrhea, an abnormal period, morning sickness, breast tenderness, urinary frequency, etc. After emergency contraception, the majority of women will have a normal period on time, but about 40% will have their period either prematurely or delayed.

Combined hormonal emergency contraceptives

Schering PC4 was licensed in 1994; its use has steadily risen since. However, after the introduction of progestogen-only emergency contraceptives its use has declined precipitously. Each tablet contains EE 50 µg and norgestrel 500 µg. The first dose of two tablets is commenced within 72 h of intercourse and the second two tablets are taken 12 h later.

Efficacy Current evidence indicates that this prevents between 57% and 74% of expected pregnancies when started within 72 h of intercourse. As with Levonelle-2, the shorter the coitus-to-treatment interval, the higher the efficacy (see Table 4.21). Hepatic enzyme-inducing agents may reduce efficacy and an IUD should be considered. In this situation, some advise an increase in the dose to two doses of three tablets each but the safety and efficacy of this have not been studied. Efficacy may also be reduced if the patient vomits within 2 h of taking either dose.

Hormonal emergency contraception will not provide ongoing contraception, and barrier methods should be advised for the rest of the cycle in which it is used. Future contraception

Table 4.21 The effect of the coitus-to-treatment interval on efficacy (World Health Organization, 1998)

Interval (h)	Levonelle-2 (progestogen-only EC)	Schering PC4 (combined hormonal EC)
≤ 24	95	77
25–48	85	36
49–72	58	31

EC, emergency contraception

should be discussed with the patient. Hormonal methods can be started with the next period.

Prescribing Schering PC4 The restrictions on use that apply to COCs do not apply to Schering PC4. In fact, the World Health Organization considers that – apart from pregnancy – there are no contraindications to its use. In the UK, it is generally accepted that severe cardiovascular disease (arterial or venous), acute focal migraine and severe liver disease are contraindications to its use.

Follow-up of patients See Progestogen-only hormonal emergency contraceptives, page 72.

Intrauterine emergency contraception

When the earliest episode of unprotected intercourse was less than five days (120 h) previously, a copper-containing IUD can be inserted as an emergency contraceptive. When the earliest episode of unprotected intercourse occurred more than five days previously, a copper-containing IUD can be inserted up to five days after the earliest calculated day of ovulation, which is day 19 of a regular 28-day cycle. Unless ongoing contraception is required, the device is usually removed with the next period or when an alternative method of contraception has been established.

Efficacy This is the most effective method of emergency contraception; therefore, unless there is a contraindication it should be the woman's decision to use it, not that of the doctor or nurse. The failure rate has been estimated to be 0.1%.

Fitting emergency IUDs Assessment for an emergency IUD is very similar to assessing someone for an IUD for long-term contraception, with the exception that long-term effects such as menorrhagia are not relevant if it is to be removed with the next menstruation.

Women requesting emergency contraception by definition have had unprotected intercourse and may be at risk of an STI. Consideration should therefore be given to screening and prophylactic prescription of appropriate antibiotics. IUDs should be fitted by doctors or nurses with appropriate training.

CONTRACEPTION IN YOUNG PEOPLE

We prescribe contraception to girls under 16 years old provided we are satisfied that the below conditions are fulfilled. These conditions are based on the test case of Gillick versus Wisbech and West Norfolk AHA (1985). The assessment of the young person's maturity was called the 'Gillick competence'. The current terminology is 'Fraser ruling competence' or 'Fraser rules', named after Lord Fraser who was one of the Law Lords who ruled in the test case.

(1) The young person understands the advice given and is sufficiently mature to appreciate what is involved in terms of the moral, social and emotional implications.

(2) We could not persuade the young person to inform her parents, nor to allow us to inform them that contraception advice is being sought.

(3) The young person would be very likely to become or to continue to be sexually active with or without contraception.

(4) Without contraception her physical and/ or mental health is likely to suffer.

(5) It is in the best interest of the young person to give contraceptive advice and/or treatment without parental consent.

Hormonal methods can be prescribed once regular menstrual cycles have been established. In our experience most young women prefer either COCs, Depo-Provera or POPs. The new implant, Implanon, is also gaining in popularity amongst younger women, who require, above all, contraception that is at the same time highly effective and 'forgettable'. We advise all young women to use condoms for prevention of STIs. Nulliparity itself is not a contraindication for use of IUD but the risks to future fertility associated with pre-existing or subsequently acquired sexually transmitted disease make the IUD a less than ideal choice for most young, nulliparous women.

Infertility

5

Nikolai Manassiev, Naim Abusheikha and John Collins

INTRODUCTION

Infertility is an important area of clinical practice. It is a common condition, affecting between 5 and 10% of married couples worldwide. A diagnosis of infertility is frequently obscure and few molecular causes are known. Specific treatment is not always effective and many couples resort to empiric treatment such as *in vitro* fertilization (IVF).

Knowledge of infertility is rapidly developing and changing. There are a growing number of textbooks devoted to infertility and the two leading journals in infertility, *Fertility and Sterility* and *Human Reproduction*, have a yearly output of over 2400 pages each. There are numerous other infertility and review journals, guidelines from professional bodies and fertility societies, and articles appearing in obstetrics and gynecology and general medical journals, not to mention the daily press, both tabloid and broadsheet. Even for the specialist it is impossible to follow them all, while for those who only seek a basic understanding of infertility it is unnecessary. Gaining a good working knowledge of infertility requires (1) an understanding of normal reproductive anatomy, physiology and pathology; (2) a good grasp of the terminology specific to infertility; and (3) exposure to patients with infertility problems under expert supervision and guidance. This chapter is designed to help the reader achieve the first two tasks.

BASIC CONCEPTS OF MALE REPRODUCTIVE ANATOMY AND PHYSIOLOGY

Brief anatomic and physiologic notes regarding the female reproductive tract have already appeared in Chapter 1. In this section a basic description of the male reproductive physiology is given.

The male reproductive system is composed of testes, genital ducts, accessory glands and penis (Figure 5.1a). The testis is about 4–5 cm long, 2–3 cm wide and over 15 ml in volume. Each testis has about 250 lobules, and each lobule is occupied by 1–4 seminiferous tubules. The tubules are twisted structures about 150–250 μm in diameter and 30–70 cm long, which end blindly. The epithelium of the tubules is where spermatogenesis occurs, and it consists of Sertoli (supportive) cells and germ cells (Figure 5.1b). The adult testis has two chief functions: production of androgens (hormonal) and production of spermatozoa (spermatogenesis).

Spermatogenesis is divided into two phases. The first phase consists of meiotic divisions of the germ cells and results in the formation of round spermatids. The second phase, termed spermiogenesis, is then devoted to a number of cytological changes leading to the transformation of the round spermatid into structurally and functionally fully developed spermatozoa (Figure 5.1c).

Spermatozoa are highly specialized cells that do not grow further or divide. The spermatozoon (Figure 5.2a) consists of a head and a tail. In the head there is a large nucleus containing the paternal DNA but very little cytoplasm. The head is a flattened ovoid 4.5–5.5 mm long and 2.5–3.5 μm wide. It has an acrosomal region, which is like a cap and covers 40–70% of it (Figure 5.2b). The acrosome contains hydrolytic enzymes like

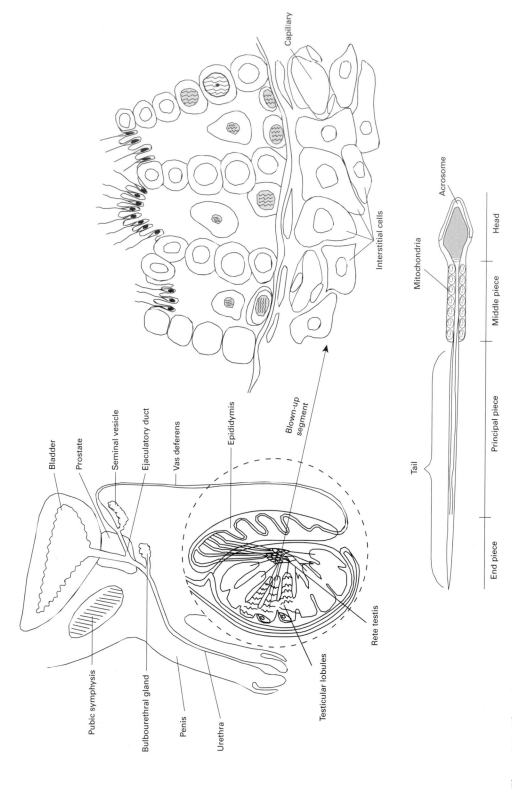

Figure 5.1 The male reproductive system. (a) Schematic representation of the male reproductive system; (b) magnification of a seminiferous tubule and interstitial tissue; (c) diagram of a spermatozoon

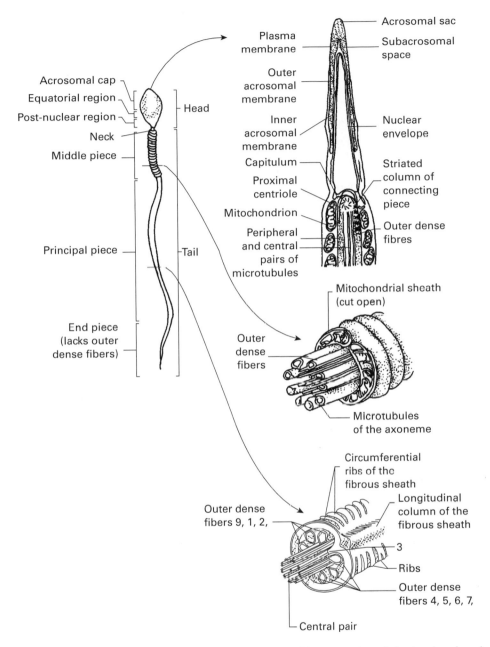

Figure 5.2 Ultrastructure of a spermatozoon. (a) Spermatozoon; (b) cross-section of the head and neck region; (c) cross-section of the middle piece; and (d) cross-section of the principal piece. Reproduced with permission from Johnson MH, Everitt BJ. *Essential Reproduction*, 2nd edn. Oxford: Blackwell Scientific Publishers, 1984:56

hyaluronidase and proacrosin which are necessary for fertilization.

The tail consists of three parts: middle piece, principal piece and end piece. The middle piece consists of several layers of mitochondria wrapped around the central axial core in a spiral fashion (Figure 5.2c). Its role is to provide the sperm with the energy that is necessary for motility. The principal piece is the longest part of the tail. It consists of nine fibrils surrounding the inner fibrils of the axial core. The whole principal piece is enclosed by a fibrous tail sheath consisting of branching and anastomosing semicircular strands or ribs (Figure 5.2d). The principal and end piece are the motile entities of the sperm. Some 40–200 million sperm are produced each day. Spermatogenesis takes 74 days on average, and the passage of sperm through the epididymis requires a further 3–12 days (8–10 weeks altogether). The production of sperm is continuous but can be disrupted by various insults, such as acute febrile illness, irradiation or medications. The role of Sertoli cells is to provide nutrients to the germ cells, to phagocytose injured/defective germ cells and debris, and to secrete androgen-binding protein, estrogen, inhibin and – in early fetal life – Mullerian-inhibiting factors. The spermatogenic compartment is under the influence of follicle-stimulating hormone (FSH) and elevated FSH levels indicate failure of this function.

The spaces between the seminiferous tubules are filled with interstitial tissue (accumulation of connective tissue, nerves, blood vessels and lymphatics). At the time of puberty, an additional cell type appears: interstitial (Leydig) cells. Leydig cells are under the influence of luteinizing hormone (LH), which stimulates them to produce testosterone. The daily testicular production rate of testosterone is 3–10 mg.

Androgens are essential for the differentiation, growth and function of the male genital ducts (epididymis) and accessory glands (seminal vesicles and prostate), male secondary sexual characteristics and sexual potency. Testosterone circulates in plasma either bound to albumin (60%) or sex hormone-binding globulin (SHBG) (38%), or unbound (2%). Estrogen, hyperthyroidism and cirrhosis raise SHBG levels and lower the available free testosterone. The opposite process occurs under the influence of excess exogenous androgens, excess growth hormone or hypothyroidism.

The semen consists of seminal fluid, which is composed of secretions from the major accessory sex glands (prostate, seminal vesicles and Cooper's glands), and sperm. The sperm are suspended in the fluid and contribute less than 10% to the total volume of the semen. Seminal fluid is not essential for fertilization as spermatozoa taken directly from the vas deferens can fertilize oocytes. However, *in vivo*, the seminal fluid fulfills an important role in providing the optimal environment for the spermatozoa. It provides a transport medium, nutritional factors (fructose, sorbitol), protective factors (buffering capacity against the acid pH of vaginal fluids) and reducing agents (ascorbic acid, hypotaurine) to protect against oxidation.

FERTILIZATION AND CONCEPTION

During coitus, the semen is deposited in the upper vagina, notably the posterior vaginal fornix. The semen rapidly coagulates due to the interaction between the prostatic enzyme and the fibrinogen-like substrate derived from the seminal vesicles. The coagulum acts as a buffer against the acidic vaginal pH and as a spermatozoal pool. Coagulation is followed by liquefaction within 10–30 min. Spermatozoa enter the cervix and the uterus within minutes of ejaculation. It is not clear how the spermatozoa travel within the uterus and tubes, but neither prostaglandins nor uterine contractions are required. It is likely that the spermatozoa move by their own propulsion and by the fluid current generated by the action of the cell cilia. The earliest that living spermatozoa can be recovered from the fallopian tubes is 2–7 h after coitus, although some dead ones may appear much sooner. At any given time, there are only several hundred spermatozoa present in the oviducts. The survival time of the gametes in the female genital tract is 28–48 h for the sperm, and 6–24 h for the oocyte.

Immediately after ejaculation, the sperm is incapable of fertilization. The ability of the sperm to attain fertilizing capacity is called capacitation. This process takes several hours, involves stripping of glycoproteins from the sperm surface and starts once the sperm are

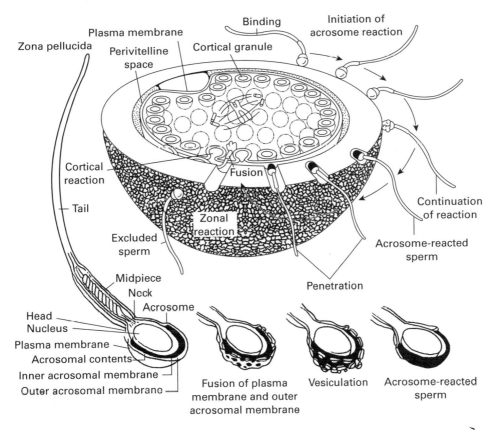

Figure 5.3 The fertilization pathway. Reproduced with permission from Wassarman PM. Fertilization in mammals. *Sci Am* 1988;259:78–84

inside the female genital tract. Capacitation has two consequences: the sperm (1) becomes hyperactive; and (2) undergoes a change in the composition of the surface membrane, paving the way for the acrosome reaction. The acrosome reaction is a process during which the surface membrane and the outer acrosomal membrane disintegrate, the content of the acrosomal vesicle leaks away and the inner acrosomal membrane becomes the only envelope of the sperm head. The acrosome reaction is triggered by a glycoprotein constituent of the zona pellucida (ZP) called ZP3, to which capacitated sperm have the ability to bind. The exposure of the inner acrosomal membrane leads to exposure of new binding sites specific for another ZP glycoprotein, called ZP2. These binding sites hold the ZP and the sperm in contact and allow the proteolytic

enzymes on the sperm head to digest a path through the ZP. The sperm passes along this path aided by forward hyperactive propulsion. ZP penetration takes about 5–20 min. The sperm eventually reaches the perivitelline space between the ZP and the oocyte membrane, where the oocyte microvilli envelop the sperm head. The fusion between the surface membrane of the oocyte and the sperm head follows, after which the sperm stops moving and its nucleus and part of the midpiece passes into the ooplasm. The first phase of fertilization, from entry into the cumulus mass to fusion, is completed (Figure 5.3).

After fusion, there is a dramatic increase in the level of free intracellular calcium, which triggers two processes lasting about 30–45 min: (1) changes in the oocyte membrane, thus preventing further sperm penetration (zona

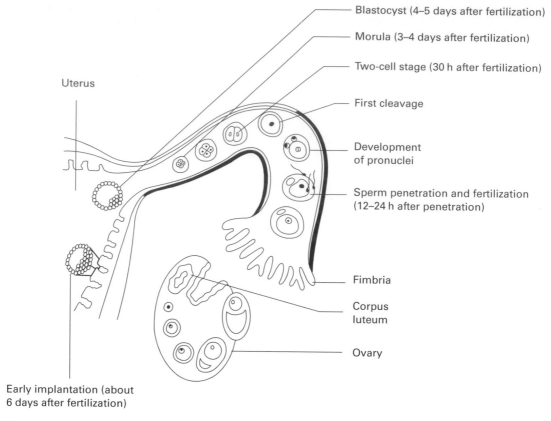

Uterus

Blastocyst (4–5 days after fertilization)

Morula (3–4 days after fertilization)

Two-cell stage (30 h after fertilization)

First cleavage

Development
of pronuclei

Sperm penetration and fertilization
(12–24 h after penetration)

Fimbria

Corpus
luteum

Ovary

Early implantation (about
6 days after fertilization)

Figure 5.4 Schematic representation of fertilization and implantation. Reproduced from Guillebaud J. *Contraception – Your Questions Answered*, 2nd edn. London: Churchill Livingstone, 1993:370, Copyright (1993), with permission from Elsevier

reaction); and (2) the oocyte, which has been arrested in the metaphase of the second meiotic division (metaphase II), is awakened. The division is completed, resulting in one haploid chromosomal set and the despatch of the second polar body. The chromosomes (22 + X) line up in a vesicular nucleus known as the female pronucleus. Meanwhile, the spermatozoon moves forward until it is in close proximity to the female pronucleus. Its nucleus becomes swollen and forms the male pronucleus. The tail becomes detached and degenerates. With the successful attainment of one maternal and one paternal haploid chromosomal set, a diploid zygote is formed and initiation of the embryo development program is started. The second fertilization phase, between fusion and the formation of the diploid zygote, lasts about 20 h. On

average, 18–24 h after fusion, the first mitotic division occurs: the one-cell zygote becomes a two-cell conceptus. The conceptus starts to divide rapidly and first forms a morula (mulberry, 8–16-cell stage), then a blastocyst (16–32-cell stage) (Figure 5.4). At blastocyst stage, the differentiation of cells destined to become a human and those destined to become placenta and membranes occurs. The conceptus becomes an embryo only after this differentiation is complete (14–18 days).

The blastocyst enters the uterine cavity and derives its nutrition from the uterine secretions while preparing for implantation. The implantation process goes through the phases of attachment and invasion. During the attachment phase (days 4–5), the ZP is lost – this process is known as 'hatching'. Early phase of implantation starts around day 6 and by day 9, the blastocyst is buried in the endometrium, which heals over it. The process of implantation is very complex and involves the exchange of messages and mutual recognition between the blastocyst and the endometrium. The implanting blastocyst starts secreting human chorionic gonadotropin (hCG), which is released in the maternal circulation and prevents luteolysis. The corpus luteum continues its endocrine function and supports the pregnancy for a total of 4–5 weeks after conception, after which the embryo is capable of synthesizing all steroid hormones required for its development.

The earliest that we can recognize a developing pregnancy is about 10–12 days post conception by means of sensitive hCG assays. So infertility (the inability to achieve pregnancy) could arise from failure of the process just described at its early stages (faulty or nonexistent germ cells) to the inability to complete the process of implantation successfully (day 9 of conception). Of course, if in the future we are able to recognize pregnancy earlier, the significance of infertility will change accordingly. It is very important to note that the terminology of infertility is different from the language of embryology. Infertility experts refer to embryo transfer (ET), when in fact it is a pre-embryo, a morula or a blastocyst which is transferred. This distinction is paramount from an ethical point of view, because many people consider manipulation of an embryo wrong. However, because of the wide usage of the term embryo in infertility we are adopting the latter in our current discussion.

THE EPIDEMIOLOGY OF INFERTILITY

For a pregnancy to occur the following steps are necessary: (1) a spermatozoon fertilizes an oocyte; (2) a viable conceptus forms; (3) the conceptus travels along the fallopian tubes; and (4) the conceptus finds a receptive endometrium where it can bury itself and continue developing. Any break in this chain of events can lead to infertility (Figure 5.5).

Infertility is treated medically as a problem affecting the couple. For simplicity, the term infertile couple is used in this chapter for heterosexual pairs engaging in procreational sexual intercourse. The normal human fecundability is about 20%, indicating that 20 out of 100 couples will conceive in any given month if engaged in unprotected sexual intercourse. In the general population it can be expected that 60% of couples will become pregnant after 6 months of regular unprotected intercourse, 85–90% after a year and about 95% after two years. Therefore a useful working definition of infertility would be 'inability to conceive within two years of unprotected intercourse'. This definition may need to be modified to 1 year in couples where the woman is over 30 years of age. For couples where the woman is over 35 years, infertility investigation is advised if no conception has taken place after 6 months of trying to conceive. The incidence of primary infertility varies between countries, and has been quoted from a low 2% in Turkey and Thailand to 21% in Zaire and 32% in Gabon. In most European countries, it is estimated to be between 3 and 7%, and about 6% in the UK and the United States. The prevalence of infertility varies: using a 1-year cut-off it is between 13 and 16%, while using a 2-year cut-off will result in about 10%. Using a 1-year cut-off some quote that one in seven couples will consult their doctors about infertility concerns and this is the figure most often used in the media and by pressure groups. Strictly speaking this may be correct, but it is misleading as it implies that one in seven couples have fertility problems, which is untrue. It is not possible to give unified prevalence figures about the causes of infertility. This is because the prevalence of various causes depends on the population studied, i.e., whether the sample comes from the general population or from primary, secondary or specialist infertility units. Causes for infertility vary between countries and within countries. According to some estimates from the primary care sector, infertility is caused by ovulatory failure (26%), male infertility (20%), tubal damage (14%), endometriosis (5%), other causes (5%) or unexplained factors (30%).

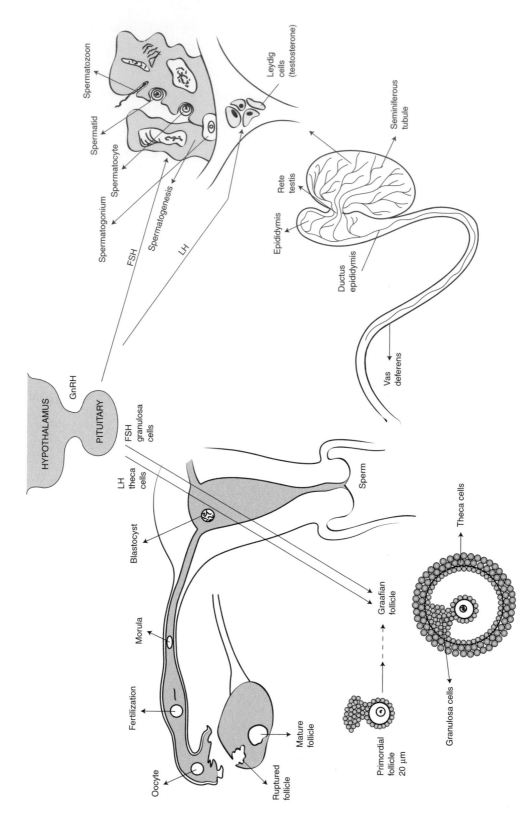

Figure 5.5 Overview of the fertilization pathway

The majority of couples are subfertile, i.e., they have relative infertility and may conceive only after a longer than normal interval. Many women become pregnant while awaiting fertility assessment and/or treatment. One estimate puts the rate at 2.02% a month and a cumulative rate of 19.9% a year. Follow-up of couples with unexplained infertility shows that 64% of women with primary and 79% of women with secondary infertility will conceive within 9 years without treatment. Sterility (absolute infertility) affects about 1–2% of the population.

CLINICAL EVALUATION AND DIAGNOSIS OF THE INFERTILE COUPLE

During the initial interview, it is important to record the age of the female partner, the duration of the infertility and to enquire if the infertility is primary or secondary, as all these factors affect the prognosis. The fourth factor correlating with prognosis is the cause of infertility. It may lie in the woman, in the man or both, and best results are achieved if the partners are evaluated together. However, single women and men may also request infertility evaluation and treatment. Infertility tests are carried out to establish the cause and to guide treatment. There are three basic infertility tests that should be done first for reasons of simplicity, cost and good correlation with conception. These are (1) semen analysis; (2) tests for tubal patency (preferably hysterosalpingography); and (3) tests for ovulation (preferably midluteum serum progesterone levels). These tests, together with any other tests deemed necessary after history and examination, should be arranged first and further management should be guided by the results.

Male factor infertility

Assessment of male infertility is based on a patient's history, physical examination, semen analysis and other specialized investigations, such as blood tests, testicular biopsy and

Table 5.1 Distribution of male infertility

Cause	%
Unexplained (no demonstrable cause)	40–50
Idiopathic*	35–40
Infection	6–7
Autoimmunity	3–4
Sexual (coital) factors	1–2
Congenital	1–2
Azoospermia	1
Endocrine	1

*Including idiopathic abnormal semen analysis and varicocele

imaging techniques. The distribution of male infertility is depicted in Table 5.1.

History and physical examination

Establishing a patient's history should include specific questions covering previous surgery in the genital area (hernia repair, scrotal trauma, torsion, cryptorchidism or late testicular descent), infections (mumps, sexually transmitted infections (STI) or urinary tract infection), metabolic diseases (diabetes, chronic renal failure or liver disease), gonadal and extragonadal neoplasia, alcohol, tobacco and recreational drugs, medications (anabolic steroids, cimetidine, sulfasalazine, phenytoin, antineoplastic agents) and occupational exposure to radiation, heat and toxic chemicals. It is also important to enquire about coital frequency and the duration of the currently encountered infertility as well as about any previous fertile periods.

Physical examination should be performed to determine general health and the extent of masculinization and general body habitus. Poor libido, impotence or lack of sexual hair growth are all suggestive of an endocrine problem. A genital examination should assess the development of epi-/hypospadias or Peyronie's disease. It is unlikely that any of these abnormalities would be unknown to the patient, but they may interfere with the intercourse or ejaculation. Scrotal content should be palpated to determine the size of the testes, which measure 4–5 cm in length.

Occasionally, cryptorchidism, anorchidia or a retractile testis may be encountered. The consistency, shape and sensitivity of the epididymis should be noted, together with any nodularity, cysts or induration. The presence of the vas deferens should be recorded. Pampiniform plexus should be palpated and varicocele should be looked for. Any other abnormalities, such as hydrocele, paratesticular cysts or hernias should be noted. Rectal examination of the prostate and the seminal vesicles may be performed if there is a history of prostatitis or STDs. We feel that the examination should be tailored individually. For example, in a patient with a negative history, a normal semen analysis and adequate masculinization it may not be necessary at all.

Semen analysis

The patient is adviced to abstain from sex for 2–3 days and asked to provide a sample by masturbation in a clean, wide-mouthed container for a laboratory examination within 2 h (normal values are given in Table 5.2). Longer abstinence increases the sperm count but adversely affects the morphology and motility. Patients should be made aware of this relationship and should be encouraged to have regular intercourse, 2–3 times a week, rather than try and time a single intercourse around the time of ovulation. If the first semen analysis is normal, then fertility is presumed and the analysis only needs to be repeated if necessary (e.g., due to changes in history, operations, etc). It should be noted that Table 5.2 lists reference values, rather than normal values. This is because there are many fertile men with sperm paramaters below the normal range. There is a 20–25% variation in the sperm count in apparently normal individuals, so if the result is abnormal, 2–3 samples should be examined within a period of 3 months. Recently, there has been much debate whether there is a trend towards a lower sperm count in the general population. Although environmental factors cannot be excluded as causes of male infertility, such a trend does not appear to exist. Intercurrent febrile illness decreases the

Table 5.2 Reference values of semen analysis. Adapted from the World Health Organization, 1992

Standard tests	Normal values
Volume	1.5–6 ml
Liquefaction	10–30 min
Sperm concentration	$\geq 20 \times 10^6$/ml
Motility	$\geq 50\%$ with forward progression > 2 (scale of 0–4)
Morphology	$\geq 30\%$ with normal forms
White blood cells	$< 1 \times 10^6$/ml
Immunobead test	$< 20\%$ spermatozoa with adherent particles
Mixed agglutination reaction test	$< 10\%$ spermatozoa with adherent particles or sperm agglutination < 2 (scale 0–3)
Optional test	
Fructose (total)	≥ 13 µmol per ejaculate

quality and/or quantity of sperm, as is exposure to lead and dibromochloropropane.

Azoospermia If azoospermia and/or a low ejaculate volume is encountered, it should be confirmed by two semen analyses subjected to centrifugation. The distinction that has to be made is between damaged spermatogenesis, obstruction and retrograde ejaculation. In order to arrive at the correct diagnosis, LH, FSH, testosterone and prolactin levels should be measured. The results of the hormonal blood tests will enable differentiation between primary hypogonadism, prolactinoma, testicular failure and germ cell failure (Table 5.3). In cases of low-volume ejaculate, measuring the semen fructose levels and examining a post-ejaculatory urine sample for sperm will help to differentiate between retrograde ejaculation and obstruction. Retrograde ejaculation is very rare but may be suspected if there is a low-volume ejaculate or a history of diabetes, multiple sclerosis, retroperitoneal lymph node dissection, bladder neck surgery or spinal cord injury. Obstruction at the level of the seminal vesicles or absence of the vesicles and vas deferens will lead to low fructose levels. Vasectomy and failed vasectomy reversal are the commonest causes of obstruction. Bilateral congenital absence of the vas is the

Table 5.3   Clinical interpretation of hormonal tests in male infertility

FSH	Testosterone	Prolactin	Interpretation
Low	Low	Low	Hypogonadotropic hypogonadism, pituitary failure/tumor
Low	Low	High	Prolactinoma (via mechanical pituitary compression), medications
High	Low	Normal	Testicular failure; if FSH > 3 × normal, consider testicular biopsy
High	Normal	Normal	Germ cell failure (Sertoli-only syndrome)
Normal	Normal	Normal	Idiopathic/obstruction/retrograde ejaculation/cryptorchidism/mumps/congenital absence of vas deferens

FSH, follicle-stimulating hormone

second commonest reason. Young syndrome – obstruction in the heads of the epididymides associated with bronchiectasias – is rare.

Germ cell failure can result from numerous causes such as cytotoxic drugs, cryptorchidism, irradiation or be idiopathic in origin (germ-cell aplasia or Sertoli-only syndrome). It is now clear that 13% of these idiopathic cases are in fact due to a Y chromosome deletion resulting in the loss of the azoospermic factor (AZFc). A testicular biopsy will facilitate the diagnosis. Germ cell aplasia is found in 10–20% of testicular biopsies performed for assessment of infertility. In such cases, the seminiferous tubules are lined with Sertoli cells and there are no germ cells. Leidig cells appear normal. In some men, areas of normal spermatogenesis may exist next to areas of germ cell aplasia. If the hormonal tests are normal and semen fructose is present, then the most likely diagnosis is an obstruction at any point between the epididymis and the point where the vas deferens joins with the seminal vesicles. Of course, it has to be bilateral such as bilateral congenital absence of the vas deferens or vasectomy. Obstruction can be confirmed by vasography, which is often performed at the time of testicular biopsy.

Oligozoospermia and other sperm defects   Isolated sperm abnormalities are uncommon, and most subfertile men have a combination of defects with a decreased sperm density, decreased motility and an increase of abnormal sperm forms (oligoasthenoteratozoospermia, OATS). Men with significant oligozoospermia ($< 5 \times 10^6$/ml) should have a hormonal evaluation and further work-up in the same way as patients with non-obstructive azoospermia, and may also require testicular biopsy. In patients with normal gonadotropins, varicocele should be ruled out if not already done. Most patients with sperm defects fall into the idiopathic category. Sperm antibody testing is indicated in cases of severe asthenospermia, but, unfortunately, there is no effective and safe medical treatment for this condition.

Sperm leukocytes   Many men thought to have leukocytes in the sperm in fact have immature sperm forms. Even in those that have true pyospermia the significance is unknown. Leukocytes and bacteria *in vitro* impair sperm motility and sperm–egg interaction, but their importance *in vivo* is uncertain. Genitourinary tract infection should be excluded by urine and prostatic fluid cultures only in symptomatic men. Routine testing for *Mycoplasma* or *Ureaplasma urealyticum* is not indicated, nor is empirical use of antibiotics. Overall, with the exception of viral orchitis or bacterial epididymitis/epididymoorchitis, infection is an uncommon cause of infertility in the developed countries.

Endocrine evaluation

Hormonal studies are indicated for the evaluation of azoospermia or severe oligospermia

Table 5.4 Indications for endocrine evaluation in men

Azoospermia
Significant oligospermia < 5×10^6/ml
Oligospermia associated with:
   low semen volume
   testicular atrophy
   gynecomastia
   demasculinization/hypoandrogenism
   decreased libido and/or impotence
   history of cryptorchidism or hypospadias

or if there is history suggestive of endocrine disorder (Table 5.4). The interpretation of the tests has already been discussed (Table 5.3 and above).

Other tests

It has been suggested that an ultrasound scan of the scrotum should be performed routinely in patients with infertility because they seem to have a higher rate of scrotal abnormalities, including testicular tumors. Perhaps this investigation should be reserved for patients with grossly abnormal semen analysis or abnormal physical examination of the scrotum. Men with undescended testes or gonadal dysgenesis are at an increased risk for testicular malignancy. Appropriate investigations should be undertaken for any man with painful testes or abnormal semen cytology. Chromosomal analysis is indicated if Klinefelter's syndrome is suspected, and tests for the cystic fibrosis gene are indicated if there is congenital bilateral absence of the vas deferens. A testicular biopsy is indicated for the assessment of severe sperm abnormalities or atypical cells in the ejaculate. Unless the physician is very confident in recognizing and treating disorders of the male urogenital system, it is best to refer the patient to an urologist with interest in andrology.

Computer-assisted semen analysis (CASA), postcoital test (cervical mucous–sperm interaction test), zona-free hamster egg penetration test, zona-binding test and reactive oxygen species assessment test have been suggested for further investigation of infertility. CASA is no better than ordinary semen analysis. The postcoital test has not been standardized and bears no correlation with pregnancy rates. The other tests mentioned above are time-consuming and expensive, have not been standardized and are mainly used for research purposes.

Treatment

Varicocele This condition is present in 25–40% of men attending infertility clinics compared with about 10–15% of men in the general population. It has been noted that the testis on the side of the varicocele has a smaller volume, which in turn is associated with a lower sperm count. Ligation of the varicocele has been shown to increase the sperm count and, if performed in young individuals, even to normalize the testicular volume. There is disagreement regarding the usefulness of varicocele repair in the treatment of infertility, but it seems reasonable that such treatment should be offered to men presenting with idiopathic low-sperm count and varicocele. Varicocele treatment shows better results the earlier it is performed, the younger the patient and the more severe the defect.

Obstruction and ejaculation disorders These cases are rare (apart from vasectomy) and are the area of expertise of urologists. Restoring the patency of the vas deferens after vasectomy is possible in over 90% of the cases, but the actual pregnancy rates are 50–60% because of the formation of antisperm antibodies. The longer the period of vasectomy, the lower the success of reversal.

Azoospermia In all patients the cause of azoospermia should be actively sought. Azoospermia due to hypogonadism (Kalman's syndrome, brain tumor, prolactinoma) may be treatable in some cases by correcting the offending factor and/or pulsatile administration of gonadotropin-releasing hormone (GnRH) analogs. In cases of obstructive azoospermia, microsurgical treatment should be considered. If this is not possible (bilateral congenital absence of the vas deferens) or not successful (reversal of vasectomy), sperm retrieval and assisted reproductive techniques should be considered. Methods for sperm retrieval are: microsurgical epididymal sperm aspiration (MESA), percutaneous epididymal sperm aspiration (PESA) and testicular sperm extraction (TESE). In idiopathic azoospermia, testicular biopsy may reveal islands of spermatogenesis with few sperm. This may allow treatment with ICSI. Donor insemination (DI) should also be offered, because it is relatively non-invasive, successful and a cheap option. The rate of livebirths per cycle is 9–14%, with a cumulative rate of 50% after 6 months. When the woman is aged ≥ 40 years, the success is much less (3–4% per cycle). Adoption may also be considered.

Oligoasthenoteratospermia Finally, we are left with the largest group of patients, those affected by oligospermia and other semen defects. The treatment options for these men are intrauterine insemination (IUI), DI, IVF-ET or ICSI. The choice depends on the severity of the defect, the effect of sperm preparation and the nature and results of any previous treatments. A summary of all treatment options is presented in Figure 5.6.

Other treatments Bromocriptine, tamoxifen, androgens and kinin-enhancing drugs (kallikrein or angiotensin-converting enzyme inhibitors) are ineffective treatments for idiopathic sperm defects/low sperm count and are not currently recommended. Antioxidant therapy with vitamin E or glutathione and mast cell blockers (tranilast) has been tested in men with idiopathic sperm abnormalities. These treatments require further evaluation before being considered as viable treatment options. Corticosteroids have been used in patients with antisperm antibodies. Reports of their effectiveness are conflicting, but evidence of their unpleasant side-effects is unambiguous. Side-effects include facial flushing, bloating, folliculitis, skin rashes, irritability, insomnia and cushingoid appearance. Several cases of aseptic

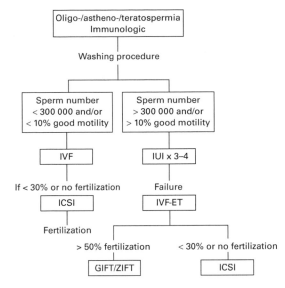

Figure 5.6 Summary for male infertility treatment. IVF, *in vitro* fertilization; IUI, intrauterine insemination; ET, embryo transfer; ICSI, intracytoplasmic sperm injection; GIFT, gamete intrafallopian transfer; ZIFT, zygote intrafallopian transfer. Reproduced from Ombelet W, Puttemans P, Bosmans E. Intrauterine insemination: a first step procedure in the algorithm of male subfertility treatment. *Hum Reprod* 1995;10(Suppl. 1):90–102, with permission of Oxford University Press

necrosis of the femoral head requiring hip replacement have been reported. Therefore, corticosteroid treatment for antisperm antibodies is currently not recommended.

Female infertility

The main causes of female infertility are disturbances in ovulation, tubal factors, endometriosis and unexplained (Table 5.5).

The actual numbers vary depending on the patient population. In areas where pelvic inflammatory disease (PID) is prevalent, tubal damage may have much higher contribution, while in areas where there is a trend towards starting a family later in life, ovarian failure may be more prevalent.

Assessment of the female patient

Points that should be covered when establishing a patient's history include PID and STDs,

Table 5.5 Main causes of female infertility

Cause	Estimated prevalence (%)
Anovulation	30–35
hyperprolactinemia	
hypogonadotrophic	
hypogonadism (low FSH)	
PCOS (normal FSH)	
ovarian failure (high FSH)	
Tubal damage	20–25
Endometriosis	5–10
Unexplained	30–35
Other causes	5

PCOS, polycystic ovary syndrome; FSH, follicle-stimulating hormone

oligo- or amenorrhea, pelvic pain, dyspareunia, galactorrhea, nutrition, body habitus, pattern of hair growth, oily skin and acne. Pelvic examination should follow next, with breast examination where indicated. It is sensible to discuss some antenatal routines and advocate the testing for rubella, and to advice the patient to increase her folic acid intake, stop smoking (if applicable) and to reduce her alcohol consumption to a minimum. Tubal patency should be checked via hysterosalpingogram (HSG), under antibiotic cover where history is suggestive of past PID and/or STD. This is normally done between days 7 and 11. The risk of infection can be minimized further by (1) cancelling the procedure if pelvic pain is present; (2) chlamydia and gonococcal screening; (3) betadine application to the cervix before the procedure. An injection of 3–5 ml of dye allows visualization of the uterine cavity and further 5 ml are injected in order to evaluate the tubal patency. The only incontrovertible proof for ovulation is pregnancy. All other tests – basal body temperature, LH peak measurement, midluteal progesterone levels, follicular disappearance on ultrasound or endometrial biopsy – only suggest that ovulation has taken place. In 95% of women with a regular and predictable cycle, ultrasound, midluteal progesterone testing and/or endometrial biopsy would be indicative of ovulation. However, since ultrasound monitoring is too labor intensive and endometrial biopsy is inconvenient, measuring midluteal progesterone levels is the standard for routine clinical practice. A luteal progesterone value above 25.6 nmol/l (8 ng/ml) is indicative of ovulation. There are commercially available kits for the detection of the LH surge in the urine. These kits show excellent correlation with ultrasound and serum progesterone levels and are used in some fertility clinics for the timing of IUI and by some patients for the timing of intercourse. Day 2–5 serum FSH/LH levels (basal values), testosterone levels and ultrasound of the pelvis should be requested if there is suspicion of anovulation, polycystic ovary sundrome (PCOS) or abnormal findings on pelvic examination. Tests for measuring thyroid function or prolactin are of no value in the absence of galactorrhea or symptoms of thyroid disease. Temperature charts, endometrial biopsy and sperm–mucus interaction tests/postcoital test are of no practical value and should be undertaken only if part of a research project. Further diagnostic testing such as laparoscopy, ultrasound sonography, saline contrast sonohysterography and hysteroscopy is undertaken if there is reason to suspect intra-abdominal (endometriosis, pelvic adhesions, fibroids) or intrauterine pathology which may need treatment (proximal tubal occlusion, resection of septum or submucosal fibroids). After the initial evaluation is done, one should be able to arrive at a reasonable diagnosis in most cases and should start planning treatment. Of course, there may be more than one pathological process present, for example endometriosis and tubal adhesions or PCOS and tubal adhesions.

Anovulation

Anovulation has many causes and is investigated by measuring prolactin and basal FSH levels. One practical approach to anovulatory infertility is to classify it according to the FSH and prolactin levels (Table 5.6).

Hyperprolactinemia Elevated prolactin levels may disrupt the cyclical release of gonadotropin-releasing hormone (GHRH),

Table 5.6 Classification of anovulation depending on follicle-stimulating hormone (FSH) and prolactin results

Low FSH levels/gonadotropic
deficiency (WHO group 1)
Pituitary tumor
Pituitary necrosis
Kallman's syndrome
Weight loss
Exercise
Medications
Stress
Idiopathic
Normal FSH (WHO group 2)

LH and FSH and lead to anovulation. Hyperprolactinemia can be caused by a microprolactinoma (< 10 mm in diameter) or prolactinoma, hypothyroidism, antipsychotic medication, drug addiction or it may be idiopathic. Prolactin levels in the blood are variable, and the test should be done in the morning (after an overnight fast) and never after a breast examination. Prolactinomas are usually treated with dopamine agonists. The most widely used drug is bromocriptine. The average dose is 2.5–5 mg/day, usually given at bedtime to avoid the effects of hypotension, should it occur. Other possible medications are lisuride, pergolide or cabergoline. Cabergoline is significantly more effective than bromocriptine in restoring normal prolactin levels and ovulatory cycles, and has a better side-effect profile with less nausea, vomiting and orthostatic hypotension. If ovulation does not occur despite normalized prolactin levels, these drugs can be combined with clomiphene. If anovulation still persists, attempts to induce ovulation can be made with FSH or pulsatile GnRH analogs. Ovulation commonly resumes within 6 months of treatment, and pregnancy rates between 34 and 70% have been reported. If after 6–8 months of ovulatory cycles pregnancy does not occur, the couple must be re-investigated. Patients with medication-induced hyperprolactinemia and drug addicts are special cases and the treatment should be undertaken jointly with a psychiatrist and/or a drug rehabilitation program.

Low follicle-stimulating hormone levels The commonest type is idiopathic, but other known causes include stress, under-nutrition, underweight and excessive exercise, eating disorders and pituitary failure. If a specific cause is found, it should be treated as necessary. In idiopathic cases or in pituitary failure, the treatment is by administration of FSH, followed by hCG in order to trigger ovulation. Pulsatile GnRH agonists is the best treatment in hypothalamic dysfunction, but it is cumbersome and involves wearing a pump that is necessary for intermittent administration.

High follicle-stimulating hormone levels Elevated basal FSH levels (12 IU/l) are found in about 5% of all women aged below 45 years and signify poor fertility prognosis. Therefore, tests should be repeated, more than once if necessary. In some cases, the cause may be identifiable (see Premature ovarian failure, page 127) but in most it is idiopathic. There is no need for ovarian biopsy to confirm the diagnosis, nor does a small increase in FSH levels form a contraindication to ovulation induction. Stimulation is a good way of establishing that ovarian failure has occurred. It is worth noting that rare cases of pregnancy have been reported, especially if the apparent ovarian failure was due to cancer treatment. However, for all practical purposes, these patients should be advised to consider adoption or attempt to get pregnant through an egg donation program.

Normal follicle-stimulating hormone levels (normogonadotropic anovulation) Most of these patients have PCOS which is responsible for approximately 73% of anovulatory infertility. The most widely accepted definition of PCOS is the association of chronic anovulation and hyperandrogenism without specific underlying diseases of the adrenal or pituitary gland.

Polycystic ovary syndrome

PCOS is characterized by a combination of a history of chronic anovulation, evidence of androgen excess and multiple subcortical ovarian cysts. PCOS has a prevalence of between 4–9% in women of reproductive age; this increases to 20% in the infertile population. The first description of PCOS was made by Stein and Leventhal[1], who in 1935 described the classic symptoms of this condition consisting of oligomenorrhea, hirsutism and obesity together with enlarged polycystic ovaries with smooth and thickened capsules. Each ovary contains multiple (8 or more) peripherally located cysts, 2–10 mm in diameter, scattered around the hyperplastic stroma. Hyperandrogenism presents clinically by acne, hirsutism and androgen-dependent alopecia, and biochemically by elevated serum levels of androgens, particularly testosterone and androstenedione. Obesity is common, as is hypersecretion of LH, but with normal or low serum levels of FSH (Table 5.7).

Ultrasound features include an increase in the amount of echogenic stroma (30% of the ovarian volume) in addition to the above pathologic features. It should be noted that polycystic ovaries (PCO) with no increase in stroma can be detected by ultrasound in up to 20% of apparently healthy women. These apparently asymptomatic women (but with a diagnosis of PCO on ultrasound) are more likely to suffer from infertility and recurrent miscarriage. If controlled ovarian hyperstimulation (COH) is undertaken, they tend to respond in a fashion similar to PCOS sufferers with multiple follicular development and a rapid rise in estradiol levels. If these patients gain weight, they tend to develop clinical features of typical PCOS.

The suspected pathogenesis of PCOS in overweight and obese women is as outlined below. High body mass index (BMI) leads to insulin hypersecretion. High insulin levels lead to decreased production of SHBG by the liver and to hyperplasia of the ovarian stroma. The hyperplastic stroma produces increased amounts of androgen. Increased total androgen

Table 5.7 Polycystic ovary syndrome

Feature	Affected (%)
Infertility	75
Hirsutism	70
Amenorrhea	50
Oligomenorrhea	40
Obesity	30
Acne	25

and decreased levels of SHBG (causing increased free androgen) lead to disruption of normal follicular growth, anovulation and high LH levels. The high LH levels additionally disrupt follicular growth and further stimulate the stroma to produce androgens and so the process is perpetuated. It is not known how PCOS develops in women with normal weight, but genetic predisposition and/or environmental insult may play a role. The diagnosis is fairly straightforward from the history, clinical examination, the ultrasound scan and the biochemical tests. Typical findings are elevated LH, normal or low FSH and elevated testosterone/androstenedione and free androgen index (testosterone/SHBG ratio). It is not necessary to perform all of the biochemical tests. FSH, LH and testosterone are commonly available and cost-effective, with specificity of 97%. Testosterone levels between 2.5 and 4.0 nmol/l (85–150 ng/dl) point towards a benign, ovarian cause of hirsutism. Higher levels should prompt further investigation to exclude adrenal hyperplasia or the presence of an androgen-secreting tumor. Late-onset adrenal hyperplasia is ruled out if the serum level of 17α-hydroxyprogesterone is below 6 nmol/l (200 ng/dl) when measured in the morning. Acanthosis nigricans, if present, reflects a more severe condition, but its presence can be reassuring because it is indicative of PCOS and not of a malignancy. It is now recognized that PCOS has numerous adverse metabolic features which put the patient at an increased risk of diabetes and cardiovascular disease (Table 5.8). It has been suggested that one of these features, i.e., insulin resistance, should be incorporated in the diagnosis. A

Table 5.8 Metabolic features of polycystic ovary syndrome

Increased waist/hip ratio
Hyperinsulinemia/insulin resistance
Insulin resistance
Increased total cholesterol
Increased LDL cholesterol
Increased triglycerides
Decreased HDL cholesterol

LDL, low-density lipoprotein; HDL, high-density lipoprotein

ratio of fasting glucose to insulin levels of < 4.5 correlates well with the results of the other biochemical tests. The majority of women with PCOS have anovulation. Chronic unopposed estrogen can increase the risk of endometrial hyperplasia and endometrial cancer. Even if anovulation is surmounted, the rate of miscarriage is double the rate observed in normal women.

Obesity is a common feature of PCOS. The more pronounced the obesity, the worse the clinical feature of the syndrome. Obesity increases the risk of high blood pressure and diabetes. If such a woman becomes pregnant, there will be a higher risk of birth defects and of a higher birth weight in her offspring; cesarean sections are also more frequent. Perinatal mortality is also increased. In obese patients with PCOS, impaired glucose tolerance is found in 30% of women and diabetes in 7.5%; in non-obese women, these figures are 10% and 1.5%, respectively. Dyslipidemia also presents at a higher rate in women with PCOS compared to normal women and increases the risk of cardiovascular disease.

Treatment General health advice to those patients who desire fertility should include weight loss, a healthy diet and exercise. Studies have shown that weight loss alone allows the resumption of ovulation in a substantial number of women. A specific treatment for anovulation is clomiphene. Clomiphene is an estrogen receptor blocker leading to the elevation of FSH which in turn promotes further follicular development and ovulation. It is usually started at 50 mg/day for 5 days from the second to the sixth day after spontaneous or induced bleeding. If there is no ovulation, the dosage should be increased by 50 mg each cycle until ovulation is induced or 250 mg/day for 5 days is reached. A 6–12 cycle treatment with ovulatory dosage of clomiphene is commonly practiced. Side effects of clomiphene include ovarian enlargement, vasomotor disturbances, visual disturbances, urticaria and alopecia, but they are not normally severe and treatment needs to be stopped in only a minority of the patients. Clomiphene is very effective and induces ovulation in 75–80% of patients, with a cumulative pregnancy rate of 80% after nine ovulatory cycles being reported. A rate of multiple pregnancy with clomiphene of up to 10% has been reported, including triplets (0.5%). Some observational studies have found a 3-fold increased risk of ovarian cancer if clomiphene was used for more than 12 cycles. If clomiphene is not effective, treatment should be discontinued after 6–9 cycles. The relatively recent understanding of the central role of insulin resistance in the pathogenesis of PCOS has prompted research on the role of insulin in the treatment of this condition. Available insulin-sensitizing drugs are metformin, rosiglitasome and pioglitasone. When administered to insulin-resistant patients, these compounds increase the responsiveness of the target tissue to insulin, thereby reducing the need for the hormone.

The best studied compound of the three is metformin. It is usually administered in doses of 500 mg tds or 850 mg bd. Metformin does not stimulate insulin production or release and when given alone does not produce hypoglycemia. Side-effects include gastrointestinal upset and in rare circumstances lactic acidosis. Metformin should not be prescribed to patients with (1) renal failure or in conditions with the potential to alter the renal function, e.g., dehydration, severe infection, shock or in the presence of intravenous iodinated contrast agent; (2) hepatic insufficiency or alcoholism; (3) cardiac or respiratory failure; or (4) for 48 h before and after surgery.

The effectiveness of metformin in restoring the normal ovulatory cycle and in improving the patient's ability to conceive has been tested in a number of controlled trials. Metformin is effective in normalizing the cycle in lean (BMI $\leq$ 24) and obese (BMI 32–35) women. The reported success rates vary between 34% after 1 month of treatment, to 78–82% after 3–6 months. The opinion on whether to use clomiphene or metformin as first-line therapy for women with PCOS and infertility is divided. Some practitioners start with metformin because it seems logical to tackle the root cause of anovulation; if there is no ovulation after 4–6 months, clomiphene is then added. Others prefer it the other way round reasoning that although metformin has been used in pregnancy without an increase in malformations or other adverse outcomes, its safety has not been fully established. A combination of metformin and clomiphene makes a substantial proportion of insulin non-responders ovulate.

Laparoscopic ovarian cyst reduction by means of cautery or laser (laparoscopic ovarian drilling) does not appear to be more effective than clomiphene and carries the risk of the anesthetic, laparoscopy, adhesion formation and the theoretical risk of premature ovarian failure. Its advantage, however, is that the risk of multiple pregnancies is avoided.

Tubal obstruction

Amongst the several causes of tubal obstruction (Table 5.9), PID is by far the most common. It is estimated that 13% of women become sterile after a single episode of PID, 36% after two and 75% after three or more. Infecundity after a single episode of PID increases with age and with severity of infection.

Tubal infertility can be diagnosed by HSG, laparoscopy or ultrasound with intrauterine infusion of sound contrast media. Initial evaluation with HSG seems reasonable if there is no indication, from the patient's history and examination, of a high infection risk. In cases of proximal tubal occlusion, filmy adhesions, sterilization, simple blockage

Table 5.9 Causes of tubal obstruction and damage

Pelvic inflammatory disease
Endometriosis
Intraligamentous fibroid(s)
Ovarian/fimbrial cysts
Sterilization

of the fimbrial end and endometriosis, surgical treatment results in a 20–60% success rate, with laparoscopic and microsurgery yielding similar results. The risk of ectopic pregnancy is about 7–9% of conceptions, and patients at risk should be seen early if they become pregnant. If surgery is unsuccessful or if the age of the patient is a consideration, IVF is the next option. Some of the patients requiring IVF for tubal-factor infertility will have hydrosalpinx. These patients seem to have worse pregnancy and livebirth rates in comparison to similar patients without hydrosalpinx. It seems that surgical removal of the hydrosalpinx improves the outcome of IVF, but the data are limited.

Endometriosis

In endometriosis endometrial tissue is found outside the uterine cavity. The etiology is unknown but several theories exist: (1) retrograde menstruation seeding endometrial fragments into the pelvis; (2) metaplasia of the celomic epithelium; (3) hematogenous or lymphatic spread; or (4) immunologic defect. The first theory is the most widely accepted.

The endometriotic lesions are variable in appearance: from non-pigmented, white, scar-like, through pinkish or red patches and papules, to typical blue-black spots resembling powder burns. The lesions vary in size, from microscopic to large chocolate-colored cysts. The incidence and prevalence in the general population is not exactly known because it is impossible and unethical to submit a large number of women to invasive procedures (laparoscopy, laparotomy). In asymptomatic women prevalence rates of 2–22% have been reported rising to 40–60% in women with dysmenorrhea. Endometriosis is more prevalent in nulliparous women.

Table 5.10 Symptoms and signs of endometriosis

Symptoms	(% affected)
Progressive dysmenorrhea	60–80
Pelvic pain	30–50
Dyspareunia	25–40
Infertility	30–40
Premenstrual staining	10–20
Painful defecation	1–2

Signs
Cul-de-sac induration
Uterosacral ligament nodularity
Fixed ovarian masses

The last 15–20 years have witnessed a sharp increase in the prevalence of endometriosis, which conspicuously coincided with the wider use of diagnostic laparoscopy. Laparoscopy allows inspection of the peritoneal surfaces from a distance of 1–2 cm with a 5–8-fold magnification, something which is not generally done during open surgery. Endometriosis should be suspected from the patient's history and clinical examination (Table 5.10). Pain is not always associated with endometriosis, even when the disease is extensive. Endometriosis may be present even if the physical examination is negative; rectovaginal examination may be performed to look for thickened endovaginal septum and/or cul-de-sac induration. Diagnosis is established by laparoscopy and the diseases is staged in four categories: minimal, mild, moderate and severe, according to the American Fertility Society scoring system. Moderate and severe endometriosis undeniably impairs fertility by interfering with ovulation, ovum pick-up by the fimbria and distorted tubal/pelvic anatomy. In minimal and mild endometriosis the link is less clear.

Treatment Treatment of endometriosis can be medical, surgical or a combination of both (surgery followed by medication). The best initial treatment for minimal and mild endometriosis is laparoscopic surgical ablation. With this kind of surgery, the combined ongoing pregnancy and livebirth rate shows a statistically significant increase (OR 1.64, 95% CI 1.05–2.57). Because of the observation that endometriosis is estrogen-dependent, suppression of ovarian function for a period of time to allow the deposits to shrink and/or disappear seems logical. However, drug-induced ovarian suppression is no more effective than placebo and has numerous side-effects. Drugs that have been tried and found to be effective for pain and disease progression, but not for infertility, are: dianazol, medroxyprogesterone acetate, gestrinone, the combined contraceptive pill and GnRH analogs. If the surgical treatment is unsuccessful, IVF should be attempted next. The results of both medical and surgical treatment for moderate and severe endometriosis are unsatisfactory and priority should be given to assisted reproductive technologies (ART).

Unexplained infertility

Unexplained infertility is present when the routine investigation of semen analysis, tubal patency and assessment of ovulation have shown no abnormality and the couple have engaged in regular sexual intercourse. It is a diagnosis of exclusion. In long-term follow-up of couples with unexplained infertility, cumulative pregnancy rates range from 27 to 79% depending on the length of infertility and whether it was primary or secondary. The prognosis worsens if the infertility is primary, if the duration is more than 3 years and with increasing age of the woman. Based on three randomized clinical trials, clomiphene has a significant but small effect: one additional pregnancy in 40 clomiphene cycles compared with untreated control cycles. Put in a different way clomiphene increases the baseline pregnancy rate in patients with long-standing unexplained infertility from 1–2% per cycle to 2–4% per cycle. Clomiphene is relatively cheap, easy to administer and has a low incidence of side-effects. Therefore, clomiphene should be considered as first-line treatment for unexplained infertility. IUI therapy also has a significant but small effect. Two well conducted trials reported a conception rate of 5–7% or one additional pregnancy in 20–25 IUI cycles compared with control cycles. The effect of gonadotropin/IUI treatment, based on the same trials was a conception rate of 9% or one additional pregnancy in 14 FSH/IUI cycles compared with control cycles. Treatment with danazol or bromo-criptine are not effective and cannot be recommended. Some studies show that treatment with gamete intrafallopian transfer (GIFT) leads to pregnancy in over 15% of cases. GIFT, however, is handicapped because (1) it is invasive; (2) it requires general anesthesia; (3) fertilization cannot be witnessed; (4) its cost is similar to IVF. In recent years IVF seems to be the treatment of choice if ovarian stimulation and IUI do not result in pregnancy after 3–6 cycles. Even with the higher pregnancy rate per cycle that is typical for IVF, however, overall pregnancy rates may not be better than with gonadotropin/IUI treatment because many couples drop out of IVF programs.

ASSISTED REPRODUCTIVE TECHNOLOGIES

Intrauterine insemination and donor insemination

The rationale behind IUI treatment is to use a sperm preparation in order to bypass the cervical mucus barrier and to increase the gamete density at the site of fertilization. As already discussed, IUI is an effective treatment in cases of abnormal semen analysis, minimal/mild endometriosis and unexplained infertility, with best results seen when it is combined with ovulation induction. There are situations when IUI with sperm from the husband is either impossible or not desirable and in such cases insemination with donor sperm (DI) is indicated (Table 5.11).

The sperm donor should have good health and no genetic abnormalities. Sperm of individuals aged between 18 and 50 years (40 years in the US) are used, and while established fertility is desirable, it is not an absolute requirement. The donor undergoes rigorous screening including medical, genetic and laboratory tests (e.g., syphilis, hepatitis B and C, HIV), physical examination and semen

Table 5.11 Indication for donor insemination

Azoospermia
Severe oligospermia
Immunologic infertility
Genetic disorder (e.g., Huntingdon's disease, hemophilia)
Non-correctable ejaculatory dysfunction (e.g., trauma, surgery, medication)
Severe Rh-isoimmunization
Females without male partners

analysis. The sperm is quarantined for 6 months and the donor is re-tested for HIV in order to exclude using sperm from infected, but not serum converted individuals. The sperm to be used for IUI and DI is first subjected to special preparation. The advantages of sperm preparation are that it removes various unwanted substances from the sperm and concentrates the most motile sperm in a small volume, which is then deposited in the uterus. Both IUI and DI can be performed as part of the natural cycle but the results are better in a stimulated cycle. Ovarian stimulation for IUI/DI is different from that for IVF treatment. The aim of the former is to induce growth of a maximum of three follicles while for the latter three is the bare minimum. This is achieved by daily injections (every other day for women with PCOS) of 75 IU of FSH starting from day 3 of the cycle. The follicular development is monitored using ultrasound, and 5000–10 000 IU of hCG is administered when the dominant follicle reaches ≥ 17–19 mm. Double insemination appears to be better than a single one. The timing of IUI/DI is 38–44 h after hCG injection if a single insemination is performed and at 20–44 h if a double insemination is performed. IUI/DI is performed by inserting a fine-bore catheter through the cervix into the uterus and 0.5 ml of the sperm preparation is then injected. There is no need for lying down afterwards and the patient can go home straight away if she so wishes. Luteal support with progesterone is advised by some, but evidence from control trials is lacking.

As discussed on page 93, in cases of unexplained or male-factor infertility, IUI is better than either natural intercourse or intracervical insemination with pregnancy rates of 5–7% per cycle, up from 2% otherwise. IUI in cycles stimulated with clomiphene or gonadotropins achieves even better results, as more oocytes are available for fertilization or subtle ovulatory defects are overcome. The best results of IUI are seen if after sperm preparation the sperm concentration is $\geq 1 \times 10^6$/ml with greater than 20% hyperactive sperm. In some centers, however, IUI is practiced with sperm concentration of $\geq 0.5 \times 10^6$/ml with greater than 10% hyperactive sperm. It seems reasonable to attempt 3–6 of clomiphene-stimulated cycles and 3–6 of FSH-stimulated cycles. If pregnancy does not follow, IVF or ICSI should be the next step. Data from the Human Fertilization and Embryology Authority (HFEA) for the year 1999–2000 show average live birth rate of 10.6% in woman aged < 38 years and 9.6% in women of all ages, per DI treatment cycle. The average figure hides considerable variations between centers with a range between 0–1.9% and 22.6–20.5%.

In vitro fertilization/intracytoplasmic sperm injection and controlled ovarian hyperstimulation

In many cases of infertility treatment IVF and ICSI is necessary. In order to improve the chances of pregnancy, more oocytes need to be made available. One way of achieving this objective is by COH. The protocol involves abolishing the normal cycle with the use of LHRH analog administration (downregulation) and recruiting a number of follicles by creating an artificial cycle using exogenous FSH and LH (stimulation). In cycles when IUI/DI is being contemplated, the aim is to recruit 2–3 follicles, but in IVF or ICSI cycles more follicles are necessary.

Downregulation

During normal cycles LHRH is released in pulses of 2–8 min every 60–90 min but after

Table 5.12 Advantages of luteinizing hormone-releasing hormone pituitary suppression

Allows recruitment of more follicles
Leads to synchronization of development
Reduces the incidence of premature luteinization
Leads to better quality oocytes and higher fertilization rates
Abolishes natural LH surge and decreases cancellations
Reduces the need for monitoring

LH, luteinizing hormone

LHRH injection treatment the levels achieved are constant and high. LHRH analog is administered daily from the mid-luteal phase of the previous cycle. LHRH administration leads to a two-phase response: (1) initial flare-up between days 2 and 4 during which preformed LH and FSH are released from the pituitary store; and (2) decrease of LH and FSH and estradiol to castrate levels by day 10–14. LHRH acts by saturating all available receptors which are then internalized in the cells with a net receptor loss. LHRH receptor production continues at a very low rate, and the receptors are immediately occupied by exogenous LHRH, so there are never enough receptors to promote a pituitary response. The suppression of the pituitary by LHRH analogs leads to several advantages: (1) recruitment of more follicles; (2) synchronization of follicle development; (3) abolition of the natural LH surge and thus premature ovulation; and (4) reduction of the need for monitoring early in the FSH administration interval (Table 5.12). Onset of menstruation indicates suppression and biochemical measurements are not normally necessary.

Recently, LHRH antagonists have been introduced into clinical practice (see section Medications used in Assisted Reproductive Technologies below)

Stimulation

Stimulation usually begins with 150 IU of FSH daily. If there is history of suboptimal response or the patient is in the older age group, the starting dosage may be 225 IU. If there is history of PCOS or previous hyperstimulation syndrome, either 150 IU are given on alternative days or 75 IU are given daily. Monitoring in the past used to be performed by measuring serum estradiol and by ultrasound, but currently it is done almost exclusively by ultrasound only. When there are three follicles over 16 mm and the leading follicle is over 18 mm and if the endometrium is over 7 mm, ovulation is triggered by 10 000 units of hCG. FSH preparations are of either recombinant or of urinary origin. Recombinant FSH (rFSH) is produced by inserting the *fsh* gene in Chinese hamster ovary cells, which on culturing start producing human FSH which can then be purified and made into a medicinal product. rFSH is 100% pure and free of urinary proteins, and the supply is relatively unlimited. Urinary FSH (uFSH) is produced by purifying the urine of menopausal women; this preparation is 99% pure, but reactions to the urinary proteins are sometimes encountered. Although rFSH is more expensive, the trend is towards its increased use. Although one meta-analysis shows that its use leads to higher pregnancy rates, one would have to use rFSH in 25 IVF cycles to achieve a single pregnancy more than in 25 uFSH cycles. Recombinant LH and hCG are now also available.

In vitro fertilization

Oocyte retrieval takes place 34–35 h after hCG administration. Egg collection is normally performed under analgesia rather than under general anesthetic. The patient is in lithotomy position and a vaginal ultrasound probe with a long puncturing needle is mounted on top and introduced transvaginally. The procedure involves puncturing each follicle individually and extracting the content by means of vacuum suction under direct ultrasound control. Cumulus complexes consisting of granulosa cells and oocyte(s) are collected and incubated for several hours. Granulosa cells are stripped and the oocytes are inseminated approximately 4 h after collection, allowing 100 000 sperm per egg. After about 16–18 h of incubation, the oocytes are observed for fertilization.

Fertilization is considered normal if two distinct pronuclei containing nucleoli are present and if the polar bodies have been extruded. Cleavage of the conceptus is evaluated after a further 24 h, and replacement of the embryo into the uterus is usually performed 48–72 h after the insemination. The quality of the embryo (pre-embryo) is estimated according to the percentage fragmentation of the cells and the clarity of the cytoplasm. The embryo should have less than 20% fragmentation and should be at the four-cell stage or more at 44–48 h. It is currently recommended that only two good-quality pre-embryos be replaced because the pregnancy rate is the same in comparison with when three or more are replaced, but the frequency of multiple pregnancy is reduced. After egg collection, GnRH administration is discontinued. However, it takes 7–11 days for the pituitary gland to recover and during this time there is insufficient production of LH to support the corpus luteum and progesterone production. Therefore, either hCG or progesterone is given as 'luteal support'. Both are equally effective. Luteal support is given for 8–12 weeks. Surplus embryos can be frozen and kept for 5 years under the current UK legislation. Embryo freezing appears to be safe but not all embryos survive the thawing, and the results of frozen embryo transfer are not as good as fresh transfer (14–17% versus 20–30% per cycle).

Intracytoplasmic sperm injection

A modification of IVF, called ICSI, was introduced in 1992. It followed previous attempts to facilitate fertilization by micromanipulation of the oocyte and sperm. Fertilization rates are very poor with IVF when the sperm count and/or motility is very low ($< 1 \times 10^6$/ml with $< 20\%$ motility), and various treatments were developed. These included: zona dissection (ZD), partial zona dissection (PZD), subzonal insemination (SUZI), all of which have been made obsolete by ICSI. ICSI was discovered accidentally when during attempted SUZI sperm was introduced into the cytoplasm of the egg, rather than into the subzonal space.

This egg was not destroyed but monitored for fertilization. When fertilization took place, a new chapter in ART was opened. ICSI is a very versatile treatment, with constantly widening indications including severe sperm defects, obstructive azoospermia and IVF failure. The main concerns about ICSI are that the selection of gametes is arbitrary and that it may perpetuate the original cause of male infertility in the male offspring. ICSI bypasses all natural sperm selection and quality control systems in the female genital tract and at the sperm–oocyte interface which might prevent defective sperm from fertilizing the oocyte. ICSI also damages the oocyte during the injection procedure, resulting in increased rates of cell degeneration. The clinical success of ICSI has overshadowed the fact that it is only 11 years old and therefore it must be practiced in conjunction with counseling, more frequent genetic testing of the father and the offspring, and long-term follow-up of any child born via ICSI. A fertilization rate of 60–65% is achieved with ICSI with 7–10% of damaged oocytes. Clinical pregnancy rates are no different from IVF and, if anything, may be better if male infertility is the only problem and the female partner is healthy. So far, ICSI appears to be safe, but the children born via ICSI are still very young. It is likely that some or all of the factors that led to infertility in the father will be inherited by some of the male offspring.

Blastocyst transfer

Recent advances in embryology have allowed us to pursue research in blastocyst transfer (day-5 transfer). With modern culture methods 40–60% of the fertilized eggs reach blastocyst stage. The principal advantages of this technique are: (1) better embryo selection and therefore better pregnancy and birth rates; (2) better synchronization between the embryo and the uterus; and (3) an improved potential to perform preimplantation diagnosis. Possible risks are that in some cases no embryo will be available for transfer and that there will be fewer embryos for cryopreservation.

At present, it is not possible to recommend blastocyst transfer.

Natural cycle IVF

IVF treatment can be carried out during the natural cycle and without COH. The cycle is monitored with serial ultrasound scans. When the dominant follicle reaches 16 mm, an ovulatory dose of hCG is given. The rest of the treatment is like conventional IVF treatment. The advantages of this technique are that it is simple, avoids the risk of OHSS and is much cheaper. The disadvantage is that the success rate is much lower than with conventional IVF. A modification of natural-cycle IVF is practiced in some clinics with much improved results. This method is called *in vitro* maturation and is used for women with PCOS. Women with amenorrhea are given progestogens to induce withdrawal bleeding. A baseline scan is performed on day 2 or 3 to exclude the possibility of ovarian cysts. Transvaginal ultrasound scans are performed on day 8 to exclude the presence of a dominant follicle. If all follicles are ≤ 10 mm, 10 000 IU of hCG are given via subcutaneous injection. Oocyte retrieval is scheduled 36 h later. In *in vitro* maturation, hCG priming increases the percentage and rate maturation of the immature oocytes. The oocytes are then cultured and checked for maturation at 24 h and at 48 h. Mature oocytes are then fertilized via ICSI and suitable embryos are transferred on day 2 or 3 after ICSI. The maturation rate is about 80%. When these mature oocytes are inseminated via ICSI, the fertilization rate is about 75%. The clinical pregnancy rate varies with the number of oocytes retrieved, and rates of 10% and 17% have been reported when 2 and ≥ 10 oocytes are harvested.

Results of *in vitro* fertilization and intracytoplasmic sperm injection

The results of infertility treatments vary from unit to unit, but in general are getting better with each year of experience. The success rate

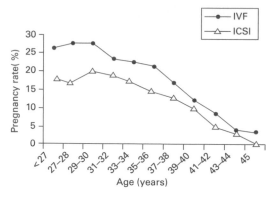

Figure 5.7 Correlation between age and pregnancy rates. IVF, *in vitro* fertilization; ICSI, intracytoplasmic sperm injection. Reproduced from *The Patients' Guide to IVF Clinics*. London: Human Fertilisation and Embryology Authority, 2000. ©Human Fertilisation and Embryology Authority

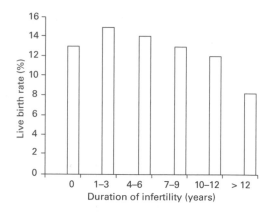

Figure 5.8 Live birth rates by duration of infertility. Data derived from the Human Fertilisation and Embryology Authority, 1999

can be measured in terms of overall pregnancy rates, pregnancy rates per treatment cycle or pregnancy rate per embryo transfer. A number of pregnancies may end with miscarriage, and therefore, the best way to measure success is by live birth rate. Other issues that need to be considered are the rate of ovarian hyperstimulation syndrome and multiple pregnancy.

The major factors that affect the chance of achieving pregnancy are the age of the woman (Figure 5.7), duration of infertility (Figure 5.8), cause of infertility and whether the infertility is primary or secondary (secondary having a better prognosis). A summary of results based on HFEA 1999 data is presented in Table 5.13 and Figure 5.9. There is considerable variation in results with some units reporting success rates about one-third of the average and others over twice the average. For women under 38 years of age there is no significant difference in pregnancy rates if two embryos are transferred instead of three but there is a reduced risk of multiple pregnancy. The miscarriage rate is about 15% of the clinical pregnancy rate and the chance of an ectopic pregnancy is approximately 2–4%. Cancellation rates of 5–20% are reported, varying between centers and between countries.

Estimation of the ovarian reserve

Some women do not respond at all to ovulation induction or respond by developing less than four follicles. These 'poor responders' are thought to have decreased 'ovarian reserve'. The term ovarian reserve describes the patient's reproductive potential in terms of ovarian follicle number and oocyte quality. Typical features are age > 35 years, basal values of FSH > 12 IU/l, LH > 5 IU/l and estradiol > 250 pmol/l (80 pg/ml). Basal FSH levels correlate very well with pregnancy rates. It has been shown that where the basal FSH level is > 12 IU/l, the fertility prognosis is poor and if the FSH level is > 20 IU/l the live birth rate is between 0 and 3%. It is currently recommended that basal FSH levels should be a screening tool in the initial infertility assessment. Some authorities advocate the clomiphene challenge test hoping to unmask patients with diminished ovarian reserve, who might not be detected by basal FSH screening alone. The value of the clomiphene test has not been fully established, but it is used by some infertility centers for women over 35 years of age prior to committing to COH. The test involves measuring basal (day 3) FSH levels, administering 100 mg of clomiphene per day on cycle days 5–9 and then measuring

Table 5.13 Live birth rates (%) from *in vitro* fertilization/intracytoplasmic sperm injection treatments

Variable	Below age 38 years	All ages	Range (all ages)
Per treatment cycle started (%)	19.6	17.4	6.0–37.0
Per egg collection (%)	21.2	19	6.9–37.8
Per embryo transfer (%)	23.6	21.1	7.4–40.7
Per frozen embryo transfer (%)	13.4	12.3	0–24.4
Abandoned treatment cycles (%)		16	
Multiple birth rate (%)		28.6	
Birth rate, twins (%)		25.5	
Birth rate, triplets (%)		3.1	

Data derived from the Human Fertilisation and Embryology Authority, 2000

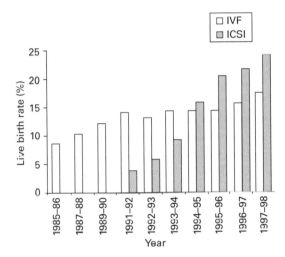

Figure 5.9 Live birth rates in *in vitro* fertilization (IVF) and intracytoplasmic sperm injection (ICSI) between 1985 and 1998. Data derived from the Human Fertilization and Embryology Authority, 1998, 1999

FSH levels again on day 10. If either of these FSH readings are abnormal (above the upper limit for the laboratory) the test result is considered abnormal.

Egg donation

There will be occasions when the use of a woman's own eggs during IVF will not be possible or desirable. Such cases arise with ovarian failure, poor-quality oocytes, poor responders, persistent IVF failure or with genetic disorders. Women in this predicament can still get pregnant if they use donor eggs. Healthy women under 35 years of age can donate eggs; these are inseminated with the sperm of the infertile women's husband and the embryo(s) is (are) transfered into the uterus of the infertile woman. The child will have a different genetic make-up from that of the woman who carries and delivers the child. The prospective donor is screened for genetic or acquired diseases in much the same way as sperm donors. Screening includes, but is not restricted to, a donor's history, blood group, infectious diseases (hepatitis B and C, HIV, syphilis, cytomegalovirus), karyotype and cystic fibrosis. The donor undergoes usual IVF treatment up to the stage of egg collection. The recipient's cycle is coordinated with HRT or GnRH agonist and HRT and the embryos are transferred to her uterus in the normal way. The live birth rate with donor eggs in the UK for the year 2000 was 21% for fresh transfers.

Medications used in assisted reproductive technologies

It can be said that modern ART is only possible because of the advances made in basic sciences and especially pharmacology. The medications used for infertility treatment can be derived from (1) natural sources, i.e. human menopausal gonadotropins; (2) be produced using recombinant technology, i.e., FSH or LH; or (3) be of purely synthetic origin, i.e., GnRH agonists/antagonists. A major new development has been the introduction of recombinant gonadotropins (FSH, LH, hCG). The recombinant technology is discussed on page 96. Recombinant FSH (r-FSH) is more expensive than urinary FSH (u-FSH). Based on current data r-FSH is more effective than u-FSH in achieving clinical pregnancy and is more cost-effective as well because less of it is used in the course of an IVF treatment cycle. Recombinant LH and r-hCG have not been used long enough to compare them to the urinary products. As mentioned earlier in the chapter, GnRH agonists are used to suppress the endogenous production of FSH and LH. This takes 7–14 days to achieve and involves initial 'flare-up' during which preformed and stored FSH and LH are released. The flare-up is used in some clinics with a so-called 'short protocol' but the pregnancy rates are lower. Therefore, the 'long protocol' is preferred. In recent years, GnRH antagonists have been developed. Unlike GnRH agonists, the antagonists do not induce an initial stimulation of gonadotropin release. The reason is that GnRH antagonists competitively bind to the GnRH receptor without receptor activation or initial stimulation. Rapid (within a few hours) and reversible suppression of gonadotropin secretion ensues. Stopping the agonist leads to a quick recovery of the pituitary function. During COH, administration of GnRH agonist is required only around the time of the expected LH surge. This allows a switch from the 'long protocol' to the 'short protocol'. In the 'short protocol' FSH is started from day 2–3 of the menstrual cycle and after 6 days GnRH antagonists are started. Both are administered for a further 4–5 days, until the day of hCG trigger. The average length of this protocol is 1–11 days and a lower total dose of FHS is required. The overall length of the COH cycle using GnRH antagonists instead of GnRH agonists is about 7–10 days less. The experience with GnRH antagonists is limited and it is not possible to tell if they are superior in terms of live birth rates or complications like OHSS. Some medications used in ART are listed in Table 5.14.

Complications of controlled ovarian hyperstimulation

Well-established complications of ovarian stimulation, whether it is used for IUI, DI, IVF or ICSI, include ovarian hyperstimulation syndrome (OHSS; Table 5.15) and multiple pregnancy.

Ovarian hyperstimulation syndrome

Ovarian hyperstimulation syndrome (OHSS) is a iatrogenic complication of gonodotropin treatment with potentially severe and even fatal consequences. Mild forms of OHSS occur in 8–10% of cycles and severe forms in 0.5–1%. The pathophysiological hallmark of OHSS is a sudden increase of vascular permeability, which results in development of extravascular exudate. Loss of fluid and protein into the 'third' space leads to a fall in the intravascular volume, loss of oncotic pressure, hemoconcentration, low urinary output and edema. A high estrogen level is a predictor and a marker of the condition, but it is not considered the direct cause. It is thought that OHSS is triggered by (1) activation of the ovarian renin–angiotensin system; and (2) secretion of vascular endothelial growth factor from the ovary. Mild and moderate OHSS presents with nausea, vomiting, lassitude, diarrhea, abdominal pain and distension. Severe forms may present with the same symptoms as above, plus ascites, hydrothorax and signs of hypovolemia and oliguria. Complications of OHSS include ovarian torsion, thromboembolism, liver dysfunction and ARDS. OHSS starts 3–8 days after the hCG injection. It should be anticipated if risk factors are present (Table 5.16), and hCG should not be administered. Prophylaxis of OHSS with intravenous infusion of albumin has not been effective.

Mild cases and some moderate cases of OHSS subside in 2–3 weeks, and can be safely

Table 5.14 Medications used in assisted reproductive technologies

Medication	Trade name	Description	Dose
Buserelin	Suprecur	Synthetic GnRH agonist 100 times more potent than the natural hormone	150 µg as a nasal spray four times a day
Nafarelin	Synarel	As above	200 µg nasal spray three times a day
Triptorelin	Decapeptyl	As above	3.0 mg SC one a day
Cetrorelix	Cetrotide	Synthetic GnRH antagonist	3.0 mg SC as a single dose or 0.25 mg/day SC
Ganirelix human	Orgalutran	As above	0.25 mg/day SC
menopausal gonadotropins (hMG)	Menogon Menopur	Purified extract from menopausal urine containing FSH and LH in a ratio of 1:1	75–225 IU SC or IM daily
Urofollitropin, high purity (HP)	Metrodin HP	Extract from menopausal urine containing FSH but virtually no LH	75–225 IU SC or IM daily
Follitropin alpha	Gonal-F	Recombinant FSH	37.5–150 IU SC daily
Follitropin beta	Puregon	As above	50–200 IU SC daily
human chorionic gonadotropin (hCG)	Choragon Pregnyl Profasi	An extract from the urine of pregnant women containing hCG secreted from the placenta	10 000 IU SC for triggering of ovulation 1500–2000 IU SC every 2–3 days for luteal support
Lutropin alpha	Luveris	Recombinant LH for use in patients with severe (< 1.2 IU/l) LH deficiency	75 IU SC daily
Progesterone	Crinone	Vaginal gel containing 8% progesterone delivering 90 mg of progesterone per application	One applicator of 8% gel daily for luteal support
	Gestone	Progesterone for injection (50 mg/ml)	50–100 mg daily IM

FSH, follicle-stimulating hormone; GnRH, gonadotropin-releasing hormone; LH, luteinizing hormone; SC, subcutaneous; IM, intramuscular

managed at home. The patients should be advised to keep well hydrated and to avoid intercourse because of the risk of ovarian rupture and adnexal torsion.

Patients who develop severe forms of OHSS need to be hospitalized. Thorough clinical examination should be performed, including weight and abdominal girth, but bimanual pressure on the ovaries should be avoided. Blood tests should include full blood count, urea and electrolytes, liver function tests and hematocrit. An ultrasound scan is useful for monitoring the size of the ovaries and ascites, if present. Treatment is by bed rest, rehydration, anti-thromboembolic stocking and perhaps subcutaneous heparin. Paracentesis (abdominocentesis) is advised if there is tense ascites which leads to abdominal

Table 5.15 Classification of ovarian hyperstimulation syndrome

Mild
Chemical
Chemical and ovarian enlargement

Moderate
Abdominal distension, nausea, vomiting, diarrhea and ovarian enlargement (5–12 cm)

Severe
Nausea, vomiting, diarrhea, abdominal distension, ascites and/or pleural effusion and ovaries > 12 cm
Hematocrit > 55%, coagulation abnormalities and/or acute renal failure

discomfort and difficulties in breathing and/or if the urinary output is poor. Severe OHSS takes 20–40 days to resolve but may

Table 5.16 Risk factors for ovarian hyperstimulation syndrome

Estradiol > 10 000–18 000 pmol/l (3000–6000 ng/dl)
> 20–25 follicles present
Thickened ovarian stroma
Ovaries > 8 cm
Fluid in the POD
Polycystic ovary syndrome
Young age (< 35 years)
Low weight
Pregnancy, especially if multiple

Table 5.17 Established maternal complications arising form assisted reproductive technologies

Allergy/erythema/injection complications
Ovarian cysts
Sedation/anesthetic complications
Vaginal bleeding
Vaginal/abdominal infection
Perforation of the bowel or iliac vessels at egg collection
Ovarian hyperstimulation syndrome
Multiple pregnancy

take longer if conception occurs. Several mortalities have been reported, including one in the UK.

The potentially very serious consequences of OHSS and the lack of specific treatment make prevention paramount. Several strategies are available and these are (1) abandoning the cycle with or without early follicular aspiration; (2) 'coasting' (stopping the gonadotropin stimulation, continuing with GnRH suppression and not administering hCG until estadiol levels decline); (3) intravenous infusion of albumin or hydroxyethyl starch at egg collection; (4) shifting the cycle to cryopreservation of the embryos; or (5) two follicular aspirations in the same cycle. Not all of these methods have been rigorously tested. The first three have been and are proven to be effective.

Multiple pregnancy

One complication of ovarian stimulation that is frequently overlooked is multiple pregnancy. The incidence of multiple pregnancy and delivery in developed countries has increased dramatically over the last 15 years. In England and Wales between 1980 and 1993, the number of twin pregnancies has increased by 25% and the number of triplet and higher-order pregnancies has more than doubled. Latest figures show that the multiple birth rate following ART is 37% in the UK and 35.5% in the US. The complications of twin and higher-order pregnancies affect the pregnancy itself, neonatal health and function in early childhood, which can make the couple forever regret seeking infertility treatment. Some complications are spontaneous abortion, preterm labor and delivery, pregnancy-induced hypertension, low birth weight, increased prevalence of congenital malformations and neurological impairments. In comparison with single pregnancies, in twins and higher-order births the perinatal mortality and the rate of cerebral palsy are both increased 5–10 times. Multiple pregnancy in IVF and ICSI cycles is almost entirely preventable and the current recommendation is to transfer only two good-quality embryos to the uterus.

Safety of assisted reproductive technologies

The issue of safety of ART relates to the mother and her offspring. Short-term complications for the mother are listed in Table 5.17. Posssible long-term complications are an increased incidence of cancer of the reproductive system. Many epidemiologic studies have looked into a possible connection between infertility treatment and cancer of the breast, ovary or uterus. So far the results have been reassuring with the exception of two early studies suggesting a possible link between ovulation induction and ovarian concer. These findings have not been confirmed by later research. However, for the moment it seems prudent to restrict the use of clomiphene to 6–9 cycles and COH to 9–12 cycles.

ART involves manipulation of the gametes and in many (perhaps most) cases bypassing the mechanisms of natural selection. Mindful of this, researchers have focused their attention on the health of children born as a result of IVF treatment. The data show that the main danger is not so much the technology itself, but the rate of multiple gestation. In summary, IVF leads to an increased rate of prematurity, low birth weight and higher rates of stillbirth and perinatal mortality (8.2% versus 6.6%). The rate of low birth weight among singletons is increased more than two-fold, from 2.5% in the general population to 6.5% after IVF/ICSI treatment. There is an increased rate of congenital malformation in IVF babies, even after excluding prematurity-related undescended testis, unstable hip and hydrocele. The malformations that occurred with higher frequency among IVF babies include spina bifida, anencephaly, hydrocephalus and esophageal atresia. In one study, major birth defects were identified in 9% of 1-year-old ART-derived babies as compared to 4.2% of naturally conceived ones. It has been reported that the risk of cerebral palsy and developmental delay is increased by 2–4 fold. However, it is important to remember that the majority of couples will not be affected and will have a healthy baby

New developments and other issues

It is beyond the scope of this book to cover the whole field of infertility. The authors would like to point out that there are many other medical, ethical and legal considerations related to infertility treatment. Here we list some of them: counseling; living with infertility; giving up fertility treatment; adoption; welfare of the child; treatment of single or gay/lesbian people; egg donation/surrogacy; cryopreservation of ovarian/testicular tissue, male/female gametes or embryos; posthumous treatment; preimplantation diagnosis; the question of when does the embryo/blastocyst become a person; fertility of the offspring; ooplasmic transfer; semi-cloning and cloning. The list will keep on expanding as medicine and society continue to evolve.

CONCLUSION

Of the specific treatments for infertility, two therapies could be considered very successful, namely gonadotropin therapy for group I (World Health Organization classification) ovulation disorders and DI for azoospermia. Although developments in the treatment of infertility have been exciting and promising, an important barrier to effective treatment is the failure to identify the molecular and membrane defects that must exist in many other cases of infertility which are unexplained or do not respond to specific treatment. Less than 50% of infertile couples are successful in having a child, and less than 5% undergo the most effective treatment for persistent infertility, which is IVF with ICSI when needed. Continuing research is necessary to reduce the cost and complexity of these treatments in order to make them more accessible.

References

Stein IF, Leventhal ML. Amenorrhoea associated with bilateral polycystic ovaries. *Am J Obstet Gynecol* 1935;21:181

Menopause, hormone replacement therapy and non-hormonal strategies

6

Nikolai Manassiev, Fergus Keating and Henry Burger

INTRODUCTION

Taken at face value, the menopause should be viewed as a normal life event. The last menses simply signifies the beginning of a new era in the woman's life cycle: the postmenopausal phase. Since all women will undergo the menopause (or die beforehand), it cannot be regarded *per se* as abnormal. The menopause marks the cessation of the female reproductive potential and is characterized by markedly decreased estrogen levels and very low progesterone levels. The roles of these hormones are quite varied. The physiologic function of progesterone appears to be confined mainly to pregnancy, but that of estrogen reaches far beyond with effects on various organs and systems; and this, coupled with the confirmed relationship between the decline in estrogen and hot flashes and sweats, has undoubtedly contributed to the definition of the menopause as an estrogen deficiency state. The menopause coincides with an age-related increase in incidence of a wide variety of potentially serious medical conditions. It is little wonder that research into the relationship, if any, between the reproductive hormones, especially estrogen, and cardiovascular disease (CVD), osteoporosis and Alzheimer's disease, for example, has attracted so much attention.

There is a tendency, however, to concentrate on the decline in estrogen levels and to describe the menopause as an 'estrogen deficiency state' or 'ovarian failure'. Although these terms can be used to define the menopause, this approach is simplistic and creates an impression of pathology. The association of the menopause with, for example,

CVD, osteoporosis and urinary incontinence gives an impression of causality, which may or may not exist. It can be argued that the menopause is only one of many factors which – together with life-style, diet, genetic predisposition and the process of aging – can be blamed for various diseases that occur with higher frequencies during the postmenopausal phase of the woman's life. Inevitably, low estrogen levels, hormonal changes and hormonal replacement figure prominently in discussions of the menopause, partly because of the causality theory and partly because there are numerous data and research studies to draw from. However, we believe in a balanced, wider, holistic approach to the menopause. We hope that in future non-hormonal strategies will figure in chapters on the menopause more prominently.

Life expectancy in the developed world has increased steadily during the twentieth century, and women commonly live more than one-third of their life in a postmenopausal state (see Table 6.1 and Figure 6.1). In the UK, 18% of the entire population comprises women over 50 years of age. There are over 10 million women in the UK in a low estrogen state (Table 6.2).

The impact of these statistics upon health resources has recently begun to be understood more fully because of the greater knowledge of the effects of estrogen deficiency on the various organ systems. As discussed below, estrogen deficiency has been linked to osteoporosis and coronary heart disease (CHD). The financial impact of osteoporosis alone has been estimated to amount to £1.7 billion

Table 6.1 Life expectancy in the UK for people of various ages

Age (years)	Men				Women			
	1911	*1971*	*1991*	*2011*	*1911*	*1971*	*1991*	*2011*
0	50.4	68.8	73.2	77.4	53.9	75.0	78.8	81.6
20	44.0	50.9	54.2	58.0	46.4	56.7	59.6	62.0
40	27.5	31.8	35.2	39.0	29.8	37.3	40.0	42.5
60	13.7	15.3	17.7	21.0	15.3	19.8	21.9	24.1
80	4.9	5.5	6.4	77.0	5.6	6.9	8.4	9.1

Data derived from the Office for National Statistics, 2003

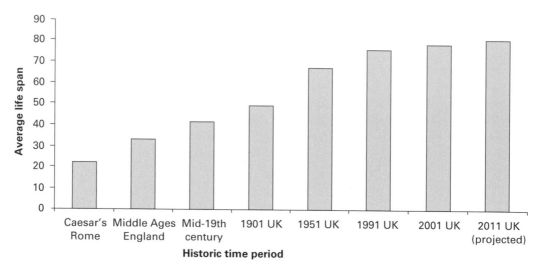

Figure 6.1 Average life span at various times in history

in the UK with some 70 000 hip fractures each year, leading to 40 premature deaths every day. CHD is the leading cause of death in women in the UK and USA: it accounts for the death of 17% of all women and 27% of women under the age of 75 years in the UK. CHD presents an enormous financial burden to the economies of the developed world, currently estimated at £10 billion per year in the UK alone (total including both direct and indirect costs to the economy). It is thus important to define precisely the link between the effects of estrogen deficiency and CHD, and preventive strategies need to be developed, if possible. This chapter presents an overview of the current understanding of hormonal and especially estrogen deficiency on various target organs, outlines the principles of hormone replacement therapy (HRT) and describes non-hormonal interventions which may improve the health of postmenopausal women.

ESTROGENS

Estrogen describes a group of steroid hormones produced primarily in the ovaries during reproductive life, but additionally in extra-gonadal sites such as adipose tissue. Estradiol is the primary estrogen during reproductive life, and is secreted by the granulosa cells of the developing follicle in response to follicle-stimulating hormone (FSH) and luteinizing hormone (LH)

Table 6.2 UK population: women aged 45–85 + (in millions)

Age band	1991	2001
45–59	4.8	5.6
60–64	1.5	1.5
65–74	2.8	2.6
75–84	1.9	2.0
85 +	0.7	0.8
Total	11.7	12.5

secretion from the anterior pituitary gland. The estradiol concentration varies throughout the menstrual cycle, with low levels in the early follicular phase (150–200 pmol/l), a peak at mid-cycle (1200–1500 pmol/l) and intermediate levels (500 pmol/l) in the luteal phase. A small amount of estrone is also produced, derived mainly by peripheral conversion of androstenedione in adipose tissue, and the ratio of estradiol:estrone in the premenopausal woman remains at around 3:1. The daily production of estradiol during the reproductive years is 0.07–0.8 mg, dependent upon the phase of the cycle. In the serum, 38% of estradiol binds to sex hormone binding globulin, a β-globulin. About 60% of estradiol binds with lower affinity to albumin. A small fraction (2–3%) remains unbound. Following the menopause, estradiol levels are commonly below 110 pmol/l, but the peripheral conversion of androstenedione to estrone increases. In the postmenopause, estradiol levels decrease more relative to estrone levels, leading to a reversal of the estradiol:estrone ratio to 1:3. Estrone becomes the primary postmenopausal estrogen, but its potency is only 1–30% compared with estradiol. Potency is measured *in vivo* and *in vitro* using a variety of assays (thus explaining the breadth of the potency range above), e.g., inducing estrus in animals, cornification (maturation) of vaginal epithelial cells, uterine weight in rodents and studying effects on cell cultures. Consequently the classic symptoms of estrogen deficiency develop, as discussed below. Endogenous estrogens are primarily metabolized in the liver where they are conjugated with glucoronide (and sulfate) to form water-soluble products, and then excreted in the bile and urine in an inactive form. In the bowel, bacteria are able to remove the glucoronide and the sulfate groups. This frees some estrogen for reabsorption which then re-enters the liver through the portal vein. This process is known as the enterohepatic cycle.

MENOPAUSE, HORMONE REPLACEMENT THERAPY AND THEIR EFFECTS ON THE BODY

Vasomotor symptoms and mood

The activity of the hypothalamus in the regulation of temperature, satiety/appetite and blood pressure, and of the limbic system in regulation of mood and psychologic well-being, seems to be influenced by estrogen. Estrogen deficiency at these specific sites in the central nervous system (CNS) is thought to be responsible for the vasomotor symptoms of hot flashes, night sweats, palpitations and mood swings experienced by over 60% of climacteric women. The hot flash of heat is a subjective sensation associated with cutaneous vasodilation and a subsequent drop in core body temperature. The hot flash may be accompanied by visible redness in the neck and face area, sweating or even panic. It is typically described as starting from somewhere around the mid-torso and moving upwards to the face. This intensely unpleasant sensation can last from seconds to minutes, usually within the range of 3–4 min. The precise mechanism underlying hot flashes is unclear, but altered thermoregulatory control from the hypothalamus is believed to be partially responsible. These manifestations of vasomotor instability show a diverse range of intensity between women, and at worse can be extremely disruptive to a woman's quality of life. The symptoms associated with the surgical menopause are more abrupt and severe and can last longer than those associated with the natural menopause. Smoking, lack of exercise and being underweight are associated with an increased risk of hot flashes. Hot flashes and their differential diagnosis are discussed in more detail in Chapter 3. Estrogen therapy is an effective treatment in reducing both the frequency and intensity of these vasomotor symptoms, and higher estrogen doses may be required in hysterectomized women. Medroxyprogesterone acetate (MPA) and norethisterone acetate (NETA) are moderately effective in treating hot flashes in women who do not want to take estrogen or in whom estrogens are contraindicated. Tibolone (synthetic compound with estrogenic, progestogenic and androgenic activity) is also effective against hot flashes and is used as an alternative to HRT. Recent randomized controlled trials produced data showing that long-term HRT may not be as safe as originally thought. This may lead to renewed interest in clonidine. The latter is moderately more affective than placebo in relieving hot flashes but it can cause sedation or dry mouth in some patients. It is licensed for treatment of hot flashes and the usual dose is two tablets of 25 mg twice a day. Phytoestrogens have been studies as a natural remedy for hot flashes as well. The results from controlled trials suggest that the effect is moderate at best and tends to be more pronounced in women with more severe hot flashes. New treatments for hot flashes are now being tested. In small controlled clinical trials, gabapentin, venlafaxine and fluoxetine were found to be more effective than placebo. However, their use in daily clinical practice is not yet established. Up to 40% of the female population experience adverse affective symptoms during the climacteric, ranging from mild anxiety states to depressive disorders, and a reduced sense of well-being. Although no definite hormonal link has been demonstrated, a beneficial effect of estrogen on quality of life measures has been demonstrated.

Urogenital system

Lower genital tract

Estrogen receptors (ERs) occur in the tissues of the vagina, urethra, bladder and pelvic floor, consistent with the fact that the lower parts of the female genital and urologic tracts share a common embryologic origin from the primitive urogenital sinus. Prolonged estrogen deficiency leads to vaginal atrophy and the classic symptoms of vaginal dryness, itching, burning and dyspareunia. Apart from the unpleasant feeling of dryness, vaginal atrophy predisposes to vaginal infection and sexual dysfunction. Estrogen replacement, whether local or systemic, has been shown to be effective in treating atrophic vaginitis, vaginal dryness and infection. Estrogen replacement leads to improved lubrication and enhancement of the pleasurable sensations experienced during sexual stimulation.

Lower urinary tract

Estrogen deficiency has been linked to urologic complaints such as frequency, nocturia, incontinence, urinary tract infections and the 'urge syndrome'. The increase in prevalence of urinary incontinence with age may be related to the menopause and diminishing estrogen levels. ERs have been demonstrated in the urinary tract. Stress incontinence arises when the urethral closure pressure is exceeded by the intravesical pressure. Estrogen may exert beneficial effects on the positive urethral closure pressure by a combination of increased urethral cell maturation and periurethral collagen production, increased blood flow and increased α-adrenoreceptor sensitivity in the urethral smooth muscle. However, recent studies have shown that the menopause has not been specifically linked to the onset of stress incontinence and may be only one of several contributing factors. Contrary to popular belief, estrogen replacement does not appear to help with stress incontinence. Estrogens may help in the urge syndrome and urge incontinence by raising the sensory threshold of the urethra and bladder. It is not clear if estrogens reduce the incidence of lower urinary tract infection.

Skin, connective tissue and cartilage

The menopause may affect all organs containing connective tissue. Estrogen and

Table 6.3 Effects of estrogen on the cardiovascular system

Beneficial effect on blood lipids and lipoproteins
Positive effect on endothelial cell function
Relaxation of the vascular smooth muscle
Decreased platelet adhesion and aggregation
Effects on coagulation and fibrinolysis
Effects on inflammatory markers
Promotion and maintenance of gynecoid body fat
   distribution
Improved glucose and insulin metabolism

androgen receptors have been found on dermal fibroblasts, and further work has demonstrated the presence of receptors in the epidermis, hair follicles, sebaceous glands and eccrine glands and vessels. Postmenopausal atrophy of the dermis results from a decrease in the dermal skin collagen content, which declines in the first five years after the menopause by up to 30%. It has been demonstrated that skin collagen content and skin thickness are increased in women on HRT compared to age-matched women on no treatment.

Middle-aged women commonly complain of polyarticular symptoms and this has fueled speculation that there may be a connection between arthritis and the menopause. The term 'menopausal arthritis' has been used to describe such complaints. ERs have been found on articular chondrocytes, but their significance is not clear. Population surveys and hospital-based studies have found that the prevalence of generalized osteoarthritis is three to ten times higher in middle-aged women than in men. Rheumatoid arthritis also shows a striking age and sex disparity. It appears earlier in women than in men and the female/male ratio is 2.3–3.7:1. HRT seems to improve arthritic symptoms, and may be a useful intervention in maintaining bone health in patients with rheumatoid arthritis who have an increased risk of osteoporosis. Although it may seem logical that HRT should be beneficial in maintaining joint health because of the abundance of ERs in connective tissue, there is no agreement on the role of HRT, if any, in these two types of arthritis.

Cardiovascular system

ERs have been demonstrated in canine peripheral and coronary arteries, in cultured rat aortic smooth muscle cells, in baboon myocardium and aorta, and in human endothelial cells. Vasodilatation in response to estrogen administration was first noted in the rabbit ear artery and later in primate coronary arteries, human umbilical and human coronary arteries. It appears that the effect of estrogen on the cardiovascular system (CVS) is complex, acting via at least eight different mechanisms that are outlined in Table 6.3.

Progesterone receptors are present in myocardium but the effect of progesterone on the CVS is less well studied. The influence of estrogen on the CVS will be discussed in further detail below.

Blood vessels

The response of vessels to estrogen is largely one of vasodilatation. Under the influence of estrogen, cardiac output increases, systemic vascular resistance decreases and blood pressure remains unchanged or falls slightly. In healthy pregnant women estrogen causes increased angiotensinogen levels and renin activity, and these lead to increased blood volume by a direct effect on volume through enhanced sodium retention. In the cerebrovascular circulation, there are gender differences. Before the menopause, cerebrovascular blood flow is greater in women than in men of the same age. Cerebrovascular blood flow is increased during pregnancy, when estrogen levels are also increased, but decreases after the menopause. Estrogen affects the reactivity of cerebral arteries to vasoactive stimuli such as serotonin.

As yet, the mechanism of estrogen's effects on the vasculature has not been fully elucidated, but several explanations have been proposed, involving either immediate or delayed effects. Immediate effects are likely to result from nitric oxide (NO) production and prostaglandin formation from the endothelium and effects on calcium channels

Table 6.4 Lipid and lipoprotein changes at the menopause

Total cholesterol	↑ by 6%
LDL	↑ by 10%
HDL	↓ by 6%
Triglycerides	↑ by 11%
Apolipoprotein B	↑
Lipoprotein (a)	↑

LDL, low-density lipoprotein; HDL, high-density lipoprotein

in the smooth muscle cells of the vessel wall. Longer-lasting effects may involve reducing angiotensin-converting enzyme activity, inhibition of smooth muscle cell proliferation and increasing the smooth muscle cell prostaglandin production by increasing prostacyclin synthetase and cyclo-oxygenase.

The normal effect of endogenous estrogen in premenopausal women, as described above, is found in postmenopausal women given physiologic doses of estrogen. Angiographic and ultrasound studies have shown enhancement in the coronary, brachial and internal iliac artery blood flows and in the cerebrovascular circulation in response to estrogen. There are reports that estrogen decreases the size of atherosclerotic plaques in the common carotid artery as measured by ultrasound scan (USS). The results of angiographic studies of coronary arteries affected by atherosclerosis are not consistent: after treatment with estrogen some studies show either no progression or reversal of the disease, while other fail to demonstrate any effect.

Lipids and lipoprotein metabolism

Premenopausal women have an overall more favorable lipid profile than men, with lower low-density lipoprotein (LDL) until the sixth decade, lower very low-density lipoprotein (VLDL) throughout life, and higher high-density lipoprotein (HDL) during postpubertal life. The differences are due to increased apolipoprotein B_{100} receptor activity in the cell membrane leading to lower LDL, more efficient clearance of VLDL, an increased rate of synthesis and a reduced clearance of HDL. Hepatic lipase activity is higher in men than in women, hence HDL is lower in men. Estrogen deficiency following the menopause is associated with adverse changes in blood lipids and lipoproteins. Many studies examining these changes have shown that there is a significant increase in total cholesterol, LDL cholesterol and triglycerides and a decrease in HDL cholesterol after adjustment for age, body mass index and smoking, though not all studies are consistent. The important HDL_2 subfraction was found to be reduced as a direct result of the menopause and there is an age-related increase of lipoprotein (a) $(L_p(a))$ after 50 (Table 6.4).

There are over 50 randomized studies on the effect of estrogen or estrogen/progestogen on lipid and lipoprotein metabolism in healthy women and in women with risk factors for (or with clinically established) coronary artery disease. Some of the studies have compared HRT with a placebo and some with statins (simvastatin). The studies have consistently demonstrated the ability of estrogen replacement therapy (ERT) to improve the cholesterol profile significantly. Typical percentage changes in lipids are given in Table 6.5. There is little difference between oral conjugated equine estrogens (CEE) and oral estradiol. Progestogens have to be added on a cyclical or continuous basis in order to protect against endometrial cancer. Progestogens have an effect on lipids that, like estrogens, depends on their chemical structure, dose, regiman and route of administration. Well designed control trials in menopausal women show that progesterone and dydrogesterone do not oppose the favorable changes in lipid metabolism induced by estrogen. The antagonism of norethisterone is minimal and the effect of levonorgestrel seems most pronounced. On this basis, it seems preferable to use HRT combinations containing dydrogesterone or norethisterone. The case of medroxyprogesterone is peculiar. In clinical controlled trials where the endpoint was changes in lipid metabolism, it

Table 6.5 Typical changes in blood lipids (%) following oral hormone replacement therapy

	Estrogen	Estrogen/progestogen
Total cholesterol	↓ 5–10	↓ 3–8
LDL	↓ 15–20	↓ 10–15
HDL	↑ 10–15	↑ 3–10
Triglycerides	↑ 20–30	↓ 10–15

LDL, low-density lipoprotein; HDL, high-density lipoprotein

showed minimal antagonizing effect on the estrogen-induced lipid changes. In trials where the end point was cardiovascular morbidity and mortality, the group treated with CEE and medroxyprogesterone fared significantly worse than those on placebo, so preparations with medroxyprogesterone are best avoided. We believe that HRT prescribing should be individualized according to the clinical condition and the nature of the dyslipidemia, to maximize the benefits and improve compliance. For example, transdermal estradiol/norethisterone may be preferable in diabetics, and continuous combined HRT is best avoided in patients with established ischemic heart disease.

Body fat distribution

Estrogen promotes and maintains the deposition of adipose tissue in the classic gynecoid pattern of postpubertal females. The ideal waist-to-hip ratio is 0.8 or less, while a ratio over 1 is abnormal. A waist circumference for women of ≤ 89 cm and for men of ≤ 102 cm is considered healthy. Based on cohort studies some researchers suggest lower number (≤ 80 cm for women and ≤ 94 cm for men). Waist-to-hip ratio measurements and dual-energy X-ray absorptiometry (DXA) measurements show that there is a post-menopausal shift in fat deposition, with a significant increase in abdominal (android) and intra-abdominal fat distribution. This may result from the decline in the estrogen:androgen ratio after the menopause. This increase in waist-to-hip ratio over time has been shown in women to be associated with a significant

increase in cardiovascular morbidity and mortality. Reversal of these unfavorable changes has been observed in randomized controlled trials of HRT.

Glucose and insulin metabolism

Estrogen deficiency leads to decreased insulin output from the pancreas, decreased insulin elimination and an increase in relative insulin resistance. While hyperglycemia itself may cause injury to the vascular endothelium, it is insulin resistance with accompanying hyperinsulinemia that may be a pivotal metabolic disturbance in the pathogenesis of CHD. Fasting blood glucose and glycated hemoglobin do not change after menopause. However, HRT decreases insulin resistance and circulating insulin levels and therefore may be beneficial.

Coagulation and fibrinolysis

It has been shown that increased levels of Factor VII and fibrinogen are risk factors for cardiovascular disease. The association of those two factors with cardiovascular death appears to be at least as strong as the association between cholesterol and cardiovascular death. The menopause itself leads to a 6% increase in the level of Factor VII and a 10% increase in fibrinogen. Orally administered 17β-estradiol decreases the level of fibrinogen. Estrogen enhances fibrinolysis in postmenopausal women by reducing plasminogen activator inhibitor-1 (PAI-1) by 50%. Little is known about the effect of the menopause on platelet function, but it appears that exogenous estrogen, or HRT, decreases platelet aggregation adenosine triphosphate release. Transdermal HRT does not appear to lead to any detrimental changes in the coagulation profile. The effects of the menopause and HRT on coagulation and fibrinolysis are summarized in Table 6.6.

The complex relationship between estrogen and coagulation is not fully understood, and the studies of coagulation are frustrated by:

Table 6.6 Menopause, HRT and coagulation and fibrinolysis

Factor	Menopause	HRT
Fibrinogen	Increase 6%	Decrease
Factor VII	Increase 7%	No change
Factor VIII/von Willebrand	Increase	Increase
Antithrombin	Increase	Decrease
Protein C	Increase	Increase
Protein S	Increase	Decrease
PAI-1	Increase	Decrease
t-PA	Decrease	Increase
Platelets	No change	Decrease aggregation

HRT, hormone replacement therapy; PAI-1, plasminogen activator inhibitor-1; t-PA, tissue plasminogen activator

(1) The use of different laboratory methods;

(2) The effect of tourniquet on sampling;

(3) Disagreement between researchers on the relative importance of coagulation variables;

(4) Difficulties in dissociating the effects of aging from the menopause;

(5) The participation of some coagulation factors in the 'acute phase response';

(6) The continuous stream of new discoveries, such as Factor V Leiden, prothrombin gene mutation, etc.;

(7) The effects of progestogens; and

(8) Differences betwen synthetic and natural estrogens, route of administration and doses.

Markers of inflamation

The current understanding is that the process of atherosclerosis is to a large extend an inflammatory process. Some blood markers of inflammation are C-reactive protein (CRP), interleukins 1 and 6, E-selection, serum amyloid protein A and adhesion molecules. These markers correlate well with the severity of CHD, the transition of stable into unstable angina and the rate of myocardial infarction (MI) and stroke. The best studied marker is CRP. The reasons for that are as follows: (1) the development of highly sensitive assays for this protein allowing the stratification of subjects within the normal range; (2) the fact that CRP levels are stable over long periods of time with the exception of the time during an acute infection (approximately 2 weeks); (3) there is no diurnal variation. CRP was found to be a strong independent predictive factor for cardiovascular events in healthy women, in women at risk of CVD and in women with established CVD. In studies, the relative risk of events for women in the highest as compared to the lowest quartile of CRP was 2.3. It is now accepted that the predictive values of CRP blood levels for cardivascular events is at least as good as that of low-density liproprotein. CRP is synthesized in the liver in response to inflammation. The signal for synthesis is usually mediated via inflammatory cytokines. The level of CRP in apparently healthy subjects correlates with the body mass index (BMI). The effect of age and menopause on CRP is not known. However, the effect of estrogen or HRT is well studied. In all studies so far 0.625 mg of CEE and 2.5 mg of MPA per day invariably lead to a substantial (80–85%) increase in CRP levels. Oral CEE increase the levels by 48–65% and transdermal estrogen by 3–10%. It is not clear if HRT stimulates hepatic synthesis of CRP or systemic inflammation or both. In any case the effect of HRT on inflammation may help explain the increase in cardiovascular events observed in HRT users during the first few years of treatment.

Summary

CVD is the main cause of death in the UK: more than one in three people (40%) die from it. The main forms of CVD are CHD and stroke. About half of all deaths are caused by CHD and about a quarter by stroke.

A 50-year-old woman has a 31% lifetime probability of developing CHD and a 17% lifetime probability of dying from CHD. This is the leading cause of death in post-menopausal women. The prevalence of CHD increases progressively with age and this may be partly due to estrogen deficiency. This assumption is biologically plausible and supported by experimental and epidemiologic evidence. A large meta-analysis of observational epidemiologic data showed a 35% reduction in the incidence of CHD and a 37% reduction in mortality from CHD in users of ERT. Moreover, this protective effect seemed greater in women who already had CHD. This wealth of encouraging data prompted a number of randomized controlled trials. The designs, endpoints and regimens were varied: some were primary prevention studies, others were secondary. Some used surrogate endpoints such as changes in coronary artery diameter, others incidence, morbidity and mortality of CHD. Oral or transdermal estradiol or CEE were used as the estrogen component either alone or as sequential or continuous combined HRT with MPA or NETA. In all but one study ERT or HRT were no better than placebo. In the one trial with positive results, new cases of CHD in the HRT group were observed. These studies are summarized in Table 6.7. What are we to make of this divergent results between observational and controlled studies? In randomized controlled trials subjects are randomly assigned to treatment and thus possible biases are minimized. In observational trials subjects who choose to take the treatment may be very different from those that do not. This fundamental methodologic difference helps to explain the results at least partially. One possible bias is the so-called 'healthy-user effect'. This means that observational trials fail to control fully for lifestyle and other health-related factors that may differ in hormone users and not-users. In observational studies subjects who choose to take ERT or HRT may be generally healthier and/or have healthier lifestyles than non-users and this imbalance may lead to an overestimation of the effect of the treatment and an underestimation of its risks. Observational studies are also susceptible to 'compliance bias'. It is known that subjects who are compliant with their treatment tend to have improved outcome even if the tretment is placebo. It is possible that hormone taking is simply a marker for better compliance with other lifestyle advice and/or treatments of CVD. It is also possible that cohort studies do not capture fully early clinical events. Let us imagine that women are enrolled in a cohort study, information is collected at baseline and update questionnaires are sent to them every 2 years. The subject is not on HRT and returns the questionnaire saying so. If she starts taking HRT shortly after that, say in 2–3 months' time, and proceeds to have an MI within the next 12–18 months for the purpose of the study she would be misclassified as a non-user having had an MI thus underestimating the hazard of the treatment. As the Women's Health Initiative (WHI) and Heart and Estrogen/Progestin Replacement Therapy Follow-up (HERS) trials show, the risk for MI early in the treatment is higher than overall. There are also biological explanations that may account for some of the discrepancy in the data between randomized controlled and observational studies. One explanation is that different regimens may have different effects. In the nurses' Health Study mose hormone users were on estrogen and those that were on estrogen/progestin were taking progestins for 10–14 days. The estrogen arm of the WHI trial continues. The implication is that estrogen may still be beneficial and that further research into different regimens and preparations is necessary. Another biological explanation is that estrogen may need to be taken early after the menopause in order to prevent the development of atherosclerosis, rather than after the establishment of atherosclerotic plaques when estrogen may raise the levels of inflammatory markers, especially CRP, and destabilize the plaques leading to clinical events. This possibility is supported by randomized controlled trials on monkeys. Whatever the explanations are for the current data on HRT and CHD we have to accept the supremacy of experimentation over observation. On the basis of this, HRT regimens cannot be prescribed for primary or secondary prevention of CHD in the populations specified in Table 6.7. However, randomized controlled trials did not show any benefit in women with established heart disease. Postmenopausal estrogen use does not affect the blood pressure and is safe to be administered to hypertensive women, when the hypertension is under control.

Osteoporosis

One in three women and one is 12 men over the age of 50 years have low bone density or osteoporosis. It is the major factor for the 70 000 hip, 50 000 wrist and 40 000 spinal fractures seen annually in the UK. As discussed earlier, postmenopausal osteoporosis represents a major public health issue. Osteoporosis has been defined as 'a disease characterized by low bone mass and micro-architectural deterioration of bone tissue, leading to enhanced bone fragility and a consequent increase in fracture risk'. The development of osteoporosis depends upon both the peak bone mass attained and its subsequent rate of loss. Peak bone mass is achieved in early adulthood and is largely (80%) genetically determined. This has been confirmed in studies comparing bone mass in twins and in studies of racial groups that have migrated. To some extent, peak bone mass is influenced by diet, exercise, alcohol consumption, smoking, drugs (e.g., corticosteroids, contraceptive pills, liver enzyme inducers), parity and the presence or absence of estrogens. Estrogens seem to have a central role in regulating bone mass and estrogen-deficient states such as anorexia nervosa, secondary amenorrhea due to strenuous

exercise, use of luteinizing hormone-releasing hormone (LHRH) analogs and the menopause have all been shown to lead to bone loss.

The development of osteoporosis results from an imbalance between bone resorption and bone formation and also depends on the peak bone mass. Loss of gonadal function and aging are the two most important factors. Starting around the fourth or fifth decade of life, men and women lose 0.3–0.5% of their bone mass every year. This is increased in women by up to ten-fold in the early years following surgical or natural menopause, due to an increase in bone turnover and bone resorption in excess of bone formation. Women may eventually lose up to 50% of their cancellous bone and 30% of their cortical bone. The speed of bone loss in later life decreases but continues inexorably into old age. The quality of bone is impaired, because the bone loss leads to disruption and perforation of the bone trabeculae which provide strength. After the trabeculae are disrupted treatment does not lead to their restoration, but merely thickens the remaining bone. The lifetime risk of osteoporotic fracture for women aged 50 is between 30 and 40% (Table 6.8).

There are several reasons for this gender difference. Women have a lower peak bone mass than men, lose more bone than men after the menopause and women fall more often than men. Women have lower muscle mass and lower agility to prevent the consequences of falls.

Currently, bone density is measured using DXA scanning. The method is accurate and reproducible with a margin of error of between 0.5 and 1%. Importantly, because many interventions increase bone density between 0.5 and 3% per year, one year of treatment may not be enough to show treatment-related changes in the bone density. Bone density varies across different ethnic groups and geographically and therefore there should be separate reference ranges for different racial groups. The mean and standard deviation (SD) are established by measuring bone density in healthy young women. One SD decrease in bone density leads to doubling of the risk of

Table 6.7 Results of studies investigating the effect of estrogen replacement therapy and hormone replacement therapy on cardiovascular disease

Study	Description	Number of participants		Mean age (years)	Mean duration of follow-up (years)	Treatment regimen	RR	CI
		Treatment	Placebo					
Herrington DM, et al. (2000)[1]	Estrogen replacement and atherosclerosis trial. Secondary prevention. Endpoint: progression of coronary atherosclerosis as measured by angiography	204	105	66	3.2	0.625 mg CEE or 0.625 mg CEE and 2.5 mg MPA for women with uterus	1.00	0.94–1.06
Waters DD, et al. (2002)[2]	WAVE. Secondary prevention. Endpoint: change in coronary artery diameter in women with atherosclerosis as measured by angiography	87	77	65.5	2.8	0.625 mg CEE or 0.625 mg CEE and 2.5 mg MPA for women with uterus	0.95	0.48–1.42
Clarke SC, et al. (2002)[3]	Papworth HRT atherosclerosis study. Secondary prevention. Endpoints: cardiac mortality, MI, unstable angina	134	121	66.5	2.6	80 µg estradiol patch or 80 µg estradiol and 100 µg NETA patch for women with uterus	1.29	0.84–1.95
Hulley S, et al. (1998)[4]	Secondary prevention. Endpoints: non-fatal MI or death	1380	1383	67	3.4	0.625 mg CEE and 2.5 mg MPA per day	0.99	0.80–1.22
Brady D, et al. (2002)[5]	HERSII. Follow up of HERS, open-label, same endpoints	1156	1165	67	6.8	As above	0.98	0.75–1.22
The ESPRIT team (2002)[6]	Secondary prevention. Endpoints: total mortality, cardiac death, re-infarction	513	504	62.5	2	2 mg oral estradiol	0.99	0.70–1.41
Rossouw JE et al. (2002)[7]	Primary prevention. Healthy women. Endpoint: incidence of non-fatal MI and CHD death	8506	8102	63	5.2	0.625 mg CEE and 2.5 mg MPA daily	1.29	1.02–1.63

RR, relative risk; CI, confidence interval; CEE, conjugated equine estrogens; MPA, medroxyprogesterone acetate; HRT, hormone replacement therapy; MI, myocardial infarction; NETA, norethisterone acetate; CHD, coronary heart disease

Table 6.8 Estimated lifetime risk of osteoporosis (%) in 50-year-old Caucasian men and women

Site	Men	Women
Hip	6	17.5
Distal forearm	2.5	16
Clinically diagnosed vertebral fracture	5	15.6
Any of the above	13.5	39.1

Data derived from Melton LJ, Atkinson EJ, O'Fallon WM, *et al.* Long-term fracture risk prediction with bone mineral measurements made at various skeletal sites. *J Bone Min Res* 1991; 6(Suppl.1):S136

fracture. The DXA scan results are expressed in two ways, as T-scores and Z-scores. Both scores are the standard deviation by which an individual bone density differs from a reference group. T-scores represent the bone density of the individual compared with the mean value of young healthy controls, while Z-scores represent the bone density of the individual compared to the mean value of their own age group. In our practice, we tend to use the T-score (young healthy controls) to assess bone density up to the age of 75. It can be argued that using the T-score results in too many women being classified with low bone density or osteoporosis. However, we think that such an argument is not in line with the measurement of the ventricular ejection fraction of the heart or the measuring of blood pressure, for example, and does little to increase the awareness in women of their bone health. Bone density and osteoporosis have been linked via the following classification from the World Health Organization (WHO):

(1) Normal bone density: mean ± 1 SD (T-score ≥ −1);

(2) Low bone mass (osteopenia): between 1 SD and 2.5 SD below the mean (−1 > T-score > −2.5);

(3) Osteoporosis: 2.5 SD below the mean (T-score ≤ −2.5);

(4) Severe osteoporosis: 2.5 SD below the mean (T-score ≤ −2.5) plus one or more fractures.

In the absence of screening for osteoporosis, a case-finding strategy is recommended.

Qualitative ultrasound is increasingly being used for bone density measurement. Studies show that there is good correlation between ultrasound assessment of the bone density and the risk of fracture. Qualitative ultrasound equipment is much cheaper than DXA scanning, requires no special room for installation and its maintenance is easier. As clinical data accumulate, it is likely that qualitative ultrasound will play a much bigger role in the future.

Another way of assessing fracture risk is by monitoring biochemical indices of bone turnover. There are two types of biochemical markers: of bone resorption and of bone formation. The markers for bone resorption are hydroxyproline and the pyridinium crosslinks with their associated peptides. The markers for bone formation are alkaline phosphatase (total and bone-specific), osteocalcin and the protocollagen propeptides of type I collagen. In a state of predominant bone resorption, the markers of resorption increase and with treatment they decrease. The markers of bone formation are low in osteoporoiss and increase with treatment. The markers of bone turnover connot be used alone for diagnosing osteoporosis but in conjuction with BMD measurement could improve fracture prediction in postmenopausal women. Bone markers are useful in monitoring the response to treatment in the early stages. Bone density measurement should be offered to those women who are at increased risk for osteoporosis (Table 6.9) or for monitoring the response to treatment.

Treatment for osteoporosis

Estrogen therapy is now well established as a prophylaxis for the prevention of osteoporotic fracture and is also effective in women with established osteoporosis. Estrogens are thought to affect the bone both directly and indirectly. The direct actions include: (1) decreasing the number of resorption pits; (2) stimulating osteoblast activity to produce more type I collagen and transforming growth factor-β; and (3) suppressing production of interleukin-1

Table 6.9 Risk factors for osteoporosis

Family history of osteoporosis
Hip fracture in first-degree relative
Low body mass index (< 19 kg/m^2)
Early menopause (under the age of 45 years)
    (prolonged periods of oligo-amenorrhea during
    the reproductive years)
Smoking
Alcoholism
Low-calcium diet
Prolonged immobilization
Rheumatoid arthritis
Chronic liver disease
Malabsorption syndromes
Hyperthyroidism
Hyperparathyroidism
Chronic steroid use (prednisolone ≥ 7.5 mg/day or
    equivalent)
Long-term (> 5 years) inhaled corticosteroids
Cushing's syndrome
Radiographic evidence of osteopenia
Previous fracture of spine or wrist with minimal trauma

Table 6.10 Antifracture activity of the most frequently used treatments of postmenopausal osteoporosis as derived from placebo-controlled randomized trials

Drug	Vertebral fracture	Hip fracture
HRT	+++	++
Alendronate	+++	++
Etidronate	++	+
Risedronate	+++	++
Parathyroid hormone	+++	0
Raloxifene	+++	0
Calcitonin	+	0
Fluoride	+	0
Vitamin D	+	0

HRT, hormone replacement therapy; +++, strong evidence; ++, good evidence; +, some evidence; 0, no evidence

and -6 and tumor necrosis factor-α. All of these actions promote bone resorption. Indirectly, estrogen is thought to: (1) reduce the level of parathyroid hormone; (2) enhance the absorption of calcium from the intestine; and (3) increase the secretion of calcitonin. The minimum daily estrogen doses associated with bone preservation in early postmenopausal women are 0.625 mg of CEE, 1 mg of estradiol and 25 µg of transdermal estradiol. Apart from estrogen, there are a number of strategies which are useful in combating this

scourge in older women, with bisphosphonates, calcium and vitamin D, weight-bearing exercise, selective estrogen receptor modulators (SERMs), calcitonin (parathyroid hormone), sodium fluoride and testosterone all being employed. There is good evidence from controlled clinical trials in favor of these treatments, and this is summarized in Table 6.10. Advice regarding osteoporosis prevention and treatment should be individualized, according to the patient's circumstances, bone density, preferences and beliefs.

The central nervous system, cognition, Alzheimer's disease and stroke

The brain is a key target organ for gonadal steroids. The gonadal steroids start exerting their effect on the CNS from the antenatal period onwards, and the effect probably continues throughout life. The CNS consequences of absolute menopausal loss of progesterone, the severe depletion of estrogen and the high levels of LH and FSH that last for 40% of the women's adult life are poorly understood. However, the permanent changes of the levels of these hormones may have bearing on both normal and pathologic brain functions.

Estrogen and the central nervous system

ERs have been demonstrated in many parts of the brain, i.e., the cortex, limbic system, hippocampus, cerebellum and hypothalamus. Estrogen is both neurotrophic and neuroprotective and able to modify the synthesis, release and metabolism of neurotransmitters in these areas. It is also believed to influence dynamic processes whereby neurites are extended, synaptic connections are formed and neuronal circuits are modeled. Studies of cross-gender hormone therapy in trans-sexual men and women imply that sex hormones exert effects on cognition, with estrogen associated with enhanced verbal fluency and testosterone with better visuo-spatial abilities. Several small observational studies in healthy women

117

during different phases of the menstrual cycle and of postmenopausal women receiving HRT have suggested that estrogen can benefit a number of skills including fine motor abilities, verbal fluency and creativity. Interventional studies seem to support beneficial effects of estrogen on verbal memory. The effect is strongest in those with severe menopausal symptoms. The magnitude of such putative estrogen effects, although modest, may nevertheless be clinically relevant.

Estrogen and Alzheimer's disease

Attention has recently been focused on the role of estrogen deficiency in cognitive function, and the link, if any, between estrogen deficiency and Alzheimer's disease. Alzheimer's disease is a neurodegenerative disease characterized by cerebral (notably cortical) atrophy, which leads to progressive memory loss, confusion, disorientation, inability to live normal everyday life independently and death. Alzheimer's disease is the commonest form of dementia, accounting for 70% of all cases of dementia. Its incidence increases with age. Its prevalence is 1% at 60 years of age, 3% at 65–74 years of age, 19% at 75–84 years of age and 30–40% in over 85-year-olds. Alzheimer's disease is the fourth leading cause of death in the USA and represents a huge burden on the healthcare system.

It is thought that Alzheimer's disease is more prevalent in women than in men (2.5:1), though some studies do not find any gender difference. The key biochemical and pathologic features of Alzheimer's disease are (1) the formation of senile plaques consisting of amyloid in brain cells; (2) neurofibrillary tangles where the leading role is played by tau protein and apolipoprotein; and (3) deficiency of the neurotransmitter acetylcholine. Experimental evidence from cell cultures and laboratory animals shows that estradiol protects the neurons from oxidative damage, enhances cholinergic nerve cell survival, promotes glucose uptake in the brain and protects against β-amyloid toxicity. Estrogens have been demonstrated to increase cholinergic

metabolism, which is positively linked to memory performance. The decline in short-term memory following the menopause may be attributable to the effects of estrogen deficiency on the neurotransmitter acetylcholine. Estrogen increases levels of acetyltransferase, the enzyme involved in acetylcholine synthesis, and thus estrogen deficiency may lead to reductions of this critical transmitter involved in many cognitive processes such as attention processing, learning and memory. Estrogen deficiency may also lead to decreased cerebral blood flow, as discussed above. If estrogen has such favorable effects on brain cells, then women using estrogen during menopause would be expected to have a lower risk of Alzheimer's disease. Epidemiologic data, however, are inconclusive. Of the longitudinal studies, the Rancho Bernardo study found no differences in Alzheimer's disease between users and non-users after 15 years of follow-up. The Manhattan Study of Aging and the Baltimore Longitudinal Study of Aging found that estrogen use was associated with a decreased risk of Alzheimer' disease after follow-up of 1–5 years and 16 years, respectively. Case-controlled studies were similarly inconclusive. A meta-analysis published in 1998 found that estrogen may have some protective effect, and noted the heterogeneity in the studies. The authors went on to conclude that estrogen cannot be recommended for the prevention or treatment of Alzheimer's disease.

More data have become available since. The Cash County Memory Study, a prospective study of incident dementia, followed a cohort of 1889 women for a mean of 3 years. It found that women who had used estrogen for 3–10 years (former users) had a markedly decreased risk of Alzheimer's disease (the longer the use, the bigger the decrease). Among current users, there was no such effect, event for those taking estrogen for over 10 years. The authors suggest that estrogen may be effective if taken early in the menopausal years. The effects of estrogen on women with Alzheimer's disease have also been studied. Four recent controlled trials published in 2002 and 2003 did not demonstrate any beneficial effect of estrogen compared to placebo. Three of the studies recruited women with mild to moderate Alzheimer's disease and used unopposed CEE 0.625–1.25 mg for 12 weeks to 1 year. In none of the studies did estrogen slow the disease progression or improve global cognitive or functional outcomes. The WHI reported on continuous combined HRT (0.625 mg of CEE plus 2.5 mg of MPA) or placebo and its effect on the incidence of dementia. It recruited 4532 women, 65 years or older and free of dementia, and the follow-up was for a mean of 4 years. The group on HRT had twice the incidence of dementia than those in the placebo group. For the moment, despite the biological plausibility and early promise, the present data indicate that estrogen cannot be recommended for either the prevention or the treatment of Alzheimer's disease. Evidence for a cause and effect relationship between estrogen deficiency and Alzheimer's disease remains inconclusive and further work will hopefully establish the precise nature of any relationship.

Estrogen and stroke

Stroke is the third leading cause of death in women, after CHD and cancer. The incidence of stroke increases with age and is higher in women than in men. Eighty percent of all strokes are caused by ischemic cerebral infarction, most often due to emboli arising from atherosclerotic changes in the major arteries supplying the brain – carotids and vertebrals. Stroke shares many risk factors with CHD: age, hypertension, smoking, diabetes and high cholesterol. Because observational studies suggested that the risk of CHD in women decreases with HRT, researchers started to look into a similar association between HRT and cerebrovascular disease and stroke. Experimental studies using Doppler ultrasound showed that the cerebral blood flow increases with estrogen administration. The thickness of atherosclerotic plaques in the carotid arteries as measured by ultrasound

seems to decrease with estrogen treatment. Despite the similarities between CHD and cerebrovascular disease, the effect of estrogen on stroke was inconsistent across studies, most showing no effect, while in some either an increased or decreased risk was noted. Results from randomized controlled trials show that (1) oral estradiol taken for secondary prevention does not have any effect on the incidence of new stroke; (2) continuous combined HRT (0.625 mg of CEE and 2.5 mg of MPA) used by menopausal women with known CHD for over 4 year did not change significantly the incidence of stroke although there were more new strokes in the treatment arm; and (3) continuous combined HRT of the same regimen as above led to a significant increase in the stroke rate when taken for an average of 5.6 years by previously healthy women. The results are summarized in Table 6.11. HRT use does not affect the incidence or severity of hemorrhagic stroke.

The conclusion is that continuous combined HRT (0.625 of CEE and 2.5 of MPA) leads to more strokes whether given to healthy women or women who suffered a previous stroke. On current evidence, estradiol seems at best neutral when taken for secondary prevention.

Colorectal cancer

Colorectal cancer has an incidence of 38 per 100 000 in England and Wales and is the second most common cancer in women in the UK. It is the third leading cause of cancer death and constitutes 15% of all cancers. Although colorectal cancer can occasionally occur at a younger age, most patients are in their sixth or seventh decade at diagnosis.

The cause of colorectal cancer is unknown but diet, genetic factors, adenomatous polyps and secondary bile acids have been implicated. The Nurses' Health Study and other cohort studies suggested that postmenopausal hormone replacement use appeared to decrease the risk of cancer by about 35%, with 'current' use affording more protection than 'past' use. The protective effect disappeared five years

Table 6.11 Estrogen replacement therapy/hormone replacement therapy and stroke

Study	Regimen and mean duration of follow-up	Treatment arm (events)	Control arm (events)	RR (CI)
Viscoli CM, et al. (2001)[8]	1 mg oral estradiol; 2.8 years	339 (99)	327 (93)	1.1 (0.8–1.4)
Hulley S, et al. (1998)[4]	0.625 mg CEE and 2.5 mg MPA; 4.1 years	1380 (82)	1383 (67)	1.23 (0.89–1.7)
Grady D, et al. (2002)[5]	0.625 mg CEE and 2.5 mg MPA; 6.8 years	1156 (59)	1165 (55)	1.09 (0.75–1.57)
Wassertheil-Smoller S, et al. (2003)[9]	0.625 mg CEE and 2.5 mg MPA; 5.6 years	8506 (151)	8102 (107)	1.31 (1.02–1.68)

CEE, conjugated equine estrogens; MPA, medroxyprogesterone acetate

Table 6.12 Absolute contraindications to hormone replacement therapy

Active
    breast cancer
    endometrial cancer
    other estrogen-dependent tumors
Acute thromboembolic disorder
Acute myocardial infarction
Undiagnosed vaginal bleeding
Undiagnosed breast mass
Severe liver disease
Severe cardiac disease

Table 6.13 Relative contraindications to hormone replacement therapy

History of
    breast cancer
    endometrial cancer
    liver disease
Previous thromboembolic disorder
Enlarging uterine fibroids
Endometriosis (recurrence)
Estrogen-dependent migraine

after discontinuation of hormone use. Possible mechanisms explaining this effect on bowel cancer include the ability of estrogen to decrease the secondary bile acid production and its ability to suppress the growth of colonic epithelial cells. These results have been since confirmed in a randomized controlled trial, the WHI study. In this trial the incidence of bowel cancer was 10 per 10 000 woman-years on treatment and 16 per 10 000 woman-years on placebo, or absolute risk reduction was 6 per 10 000 woman-years and relative risk reduction was 37%.

Gums, teeth, wound healing and postural balance

The effects of the menopause and HRT on oral health, wound healing and balance are less well studied. The data so far show that ERT prevents tooth loss and gum disease, enhances wound healing and improves postural balance in postmenopausal women.

CONTRAINDICATIONS AND RISKS OF HORMONE REPLACEMENT THERAPY

There are remarkably few absolute (Table 6.12) or relative contraindications to HRT (Table 6.13).

There are many other contraindications and special precautions to be found on the HRT prescribing data sheets. Usually these are included on the basis of data from studies of the oral contraceptives or from purely theoretical considerations. In the view of most experts HRT is not contraindicated for those conditions listed in Table 6.14. This view was endorsed by the British Menopause Society in a recent publication.

Table 6.14 Conditions no longer considered contraindications to hormone replacement therapy

Controlled hypertension
Coronary heart disease*
Varicose veins
History of superficial thrombophlebitis
Otosclerosis
Malignant melanoma
History of cervical cancer
History of ovarian cancer
Benign breast disease

Certain regimens may be contraindicated. Data derived from Rees M, Purdie DW. *Management of the Menopause. The Handbook of the British Menopause Society*. London: BMS Publications, 1999:39

Risks of hormone replacement therapy

Breast cancer

The widely discussed possibility that HRT leads to an increase in the risk of breast cancer has been responsible for much of the controversy surrounding the treatment. The data available from observational studies are widely disparate. A recent meta-analysis of 90% of the available world breast cancer data (over 52 700 cases and 108 000 controls) has to a large extent overridden the individual studies and has made counseling women easier (Table 6.15). The study has estimated the background risk of breast cancer incidence in 50- to 70-year-old women at 45/1000 women and has shown significant increases in breast cancer incidence among HRT users. However, this increased risk returned to background levels within five years after discontinuation of therapy. The study reported that body mass index is an independent risk factor for breast cancer: the higher the body mass index, the higher the risk. An important but often overlooked finding was that the excess risk of breast cancer attributed to HRT was confined to women with a BMI of less than 25 kg/m². The two findings above have subsequently been confirmed in another study. The increase in the relative risk of breast cancer with HRT can be calculated for each year of HRT use. It would seem prudent, therefore, to assess both the potential benefit of using HRT and the risk of developing breast cancer in the case of each individual woman. The addition of a progestogen does not decrease the risk of breast cancer and if anything it may lead to slight increase in the risk. HRT increases the density of the breast tissue and may decrease the sensitivity of screening mammography. The Nurses' Health Study reported an increase in risk of dying from breast cancer among users in comparison to non-users, but many studies have reported exactly the opposite. It is conceivable that HRT use may lead to lower death rate because (1) women taking HRT may be healthier at the outset, (2) HRT users tend to have lower all-cause mortality than non-users, and (3) breast cancer striking women on HRT may behave differently with less incidence of lymph node involvement and distant spread. The WHI trial had a secondary endpoint, i.e., the incidence of breast cancer. There was a 26% increase (38 versus 30 per 10 000 woman-years) in the HRT group and no difference in the risk of *in situ* cancer or breast cancer mortality between the groups.

Endometrial hyperplasia and endometrial cancer

Unopposed use of estrogen increases the risk of endometrial hyperplasia and endometrial carcinoma. The longer the duration of treatment and the higher the estrogen dosage, the higher the risk. The incidence of endometrial hyperplasia is 20, 50 and 62% after one, two and three years' use of 0.625 mg/day of CEE, whereas the background rate of this condition is between 0.5 and 2% a year. Similarly, there is a three- to ten-fold increase in the incidence of endometrial cancer with unopposed estrogen, depending on the duration of use. Sufficient doses of progestogen, given cyclically for 12–14 days, largely eliminate the risk of endometrial hyperplasia and cancer, but there are studies suggesting that the risk is not completely abolished. Continuous combined HRT offers the best endometrial protection and may even decrease the risks of endometrial

Table 6.15 Relative and absolute risks of breast cancer with hormone replacement therapy (HRT)

Current HRT users: RR = 1.023 per year of use
Long use (~ 11 yrs): RR = 1.35
For each year of delayed menopause: RR = 1.028

Absolute risk: age 50–70

Year]s of use	Cases per 1000	Extra cases per 1000 HRT users
Never used	45	0
5 years of use	47	2
10 years of use	51	6
15 years of use	57	12

RR, relative risk. Data derived from Collaborative Group on Hormonal Factors in Breast Cancer. Breast cancer and hormone replacement therapy: collaborative reanalysis of data from 51 epidemiological studies of 52 705 women with breast cancer and 108 411 women without breast cancer. *Lancet* 1997;350:1047–59

hyperplasia and carcinoma to below those seen in an untreated population. Therefore, in women with a uterus, progestogens must always be prescribed for at least 12–14 days every month or continuously. Recommended oral doses for endometrial protection in sequential regimens are:

(1)   Norethisterone: 0.7–2.5 mg;

(2)   Norgestrel: 75–150 mg;

(3)   Dydrogesterone: 10–20 mg;

(4)   Medroxyprogesterone: 5–10 mg.

Endometrial protection can be achieved by inserting a levonorgestrel-releasing intrauterine device (Mirena) or by intravaginal progesterone administration (Crinone gel). Progesterone pessaries (Cyclogest) and oral micronized progesterone (Utrogestan) can also be used, but are not licensed for this indication in the UK. With monthly sequential HRT, 70–90% of women will have vaginal bleeding, which commonly starts after the ninth day of progestogen and should be no heavier than a normal period. With continuous combined HRT, about 50–80% of women will stop bleeding after 12 months of treatment. Irregular bleeding associated with HRT use is a common cause of anxiety among women and their doctors and often leads to discontinuation of

HRT. The initial approach should include assessment of the problem via history taking and clinical examination. Although the causes of vaginal bleeding are numerous (Table 6.16), in most cases the bleeding is caused by HRT and not by disease, or can be due to poor compliance, altered gastrointestinal absorption or a drug interaction.

When pathology is absent, a change of regimen, medication or dose may be enough to eliminate the problem. However, endometrial assessment is advised if there is:

(1)   Heavy withdrawal bleeding;

(2)   Prolonged withdrawal bleeding;

(3)   Breakthrough bleeding for two or more consecutive cycles;

(4)   Bleeding in women on continuous combined HRT starting after a period of amenorrhea;

(5)   Bleeding continuing for six months after starting continuous combined HRT.

Endometrial assessment is by means of vaginal USS and endometrial biopsy, but occasionally hysteroscopy may be necessary. On USS, endometrial thickness, double layer, of 4 mm or less excludes endometrial carcinoma. Endometrial biopsy is an outpatient

Table 6.16   Causes of postmenopausal bleeding

(1) *Malignant lesions*
    (a) Endometrium
          cancer
          endometrial hyperplasia
    (b) Other malignancy of the genital tract
          vagina
          vulva
          uterine sarcoma
          rarely associated with fallopian tube or ovarian cancer

(2) *Non-malignant lesions of the genital tract*
      atrophic endometrium, vagina and/or cervix
      polyps
      fibroids
      endometritis, cervicitis
      vulvar lesions
      trauma
      parasitic infections

(3) *Other sources of bleeding outside the genital tract*
      urethral (urologic system: urethral cruncle, cystitis, etc.)
      rectal (and intestinal diseases): hemorrhoids, rectal neoplasm, etc.

Table 6.17   Hormone replacement therapy and deep venous thrombosis

Risk	Non-users	Users
RR for DVT	1.0	2.1–3.6
RR for PE	1.0	2.1
Absolute for DVT	9–13/100 000	26–35/100 000
Absolute for PE	< 1/100 000	2–3/100 000

RR, relative risk; PE, pulmonary embolism

procedure and commonly used devices are Pipelle and Vabra. Its limitations are that it is a blind procedure, samples between 4 and 40% (Vabra) of the endometrial surface, may miss a polyp and can cause discomfort or pain. Sometimes the procedure is not possible to perform because of pain or tight cervical sclerosis, or does not provide an adequate sample. In those cases, hysteroscopy and dilatation and curettage (D&C) should be considered. For women on sequential therapy, the ultrasound should be performed immediately after the withdrawal bleeding because the endometrial thickness depends on the phase of the therapy. If the ultrasound scan shows an endometrial thickness < 4 mm, further assessment may not be necessary. If the endometrial thickness is > 4 mm, an endometrial biopsy should be performed. Ultrasound is a very good technique for assessing women on continuous combined HRT. Endometrial biopsy in such patients may not yield any sample.

Thromboembolism

The effects of HRT on hemostasis are complex, and recent observational and randomized controlled studies have shown a two- to three-fold increase in risk of venous thromboembolism (VTE) in current users of HRT (Table 6.17). Deep venous thrombosis (DVT) is the commonest form of VTE and in 10% of cases it may lead to pulmonary embolism (PE). The mortality of PE is 1–2%.

A substantial proportion of thromboembolic episodes occur in women with disorders of coagulation, for example deficiency of antithrombin, protein C or protein S, APC resistance/Factor V Leiden, or G20210A prothrombin gene mutation. These conditions tend to run in families and are known as familial thrombophilias. The prevalence of thrombophilia in healthy individuals and in those with VTE is summarized in Table 6.18.

Table 6.18 Prevalence of thrombophilia in healthy individuals and those with venous thromboembolism (VTE)

Thrombophilia factor	Prevalence in healthy population (%)	Prevalence in patients with VTE (%)	RR of thrombosis if thrombophilia factor present
Factor V Leiden	5	40	5
Prothrombin G 20210A gene mutation	3	6–16	2–5
Protein S deficiency	2	4	2
Protein C deficiency	0.3	3–5	>10
Antithrombin deficiency	0.02	1	25–50

Table 6.19 Features suggestive of familial thrombophilia

Family history of VTE

First episode at an early age (< 45 years)

Recurrent VTE

Unusual site of thrombosis, e.g., cerebral, mesenteric

Thrombosis during pregnancy or puerperium or use of COC or HRT

Spontaneous venous thrombosis without environmental or acquired risk factor

Recurrent superficial thrombophlebitis

Pulmonary embolism

Unexplained stillbirth

Unexplained spontaneous abortions (≥ 3)

VTE, venous thromboembolism; COC, combined oral contraceptive; HRT, hormone replacement therapy

If there are historic features suggestive of thrombophilias (Table 6.19), a coagulation screen should be performed before prescribing HRT. In women with thrombophilia, HRT is contraindicated. In cases where long immobilization is expected, such as fracture or peri-operatively, HRT needs to be terminated. In cases of long distance travel the standard advice is to keep well hydrated, move around or exercise the legs frequently and wear compressive hosiery.

Hormone replacement therapy and endometriosis

Women with a history of endometriosis often require extensive counseling regarding the risk of recurrence with HRT. They may be reassured that such a risk is mainly theoretical and rather remote. Indeed, the current accepted medical treatment for endometriosis is LHRH analogs with add-back HRT.

Hormone replacement therapy and fibroids

There is a theoretical possibility that HRT may lead to enlargement of fibroids, because they are hormone- and, especially, estrogen-dependent. Evidence for this fact is that fibroids commonly enlarge during pregnancy and that treatment of fibroids with LHRH analogs is effective and is often practiced before surgical intervention. However, we have not found this to be a problem and in our clinic we reassure women that HRT is unlikely to lead to recurrence or enlargement of fibroids. We recommend that fibroids are monitored by USS, twice in the first year of HRT and then yearly.

PRESCRIBING HORMONE REPLACEMENT THERAPY

Compliance

Prescribing HRT is complicated by the difficulties in persuading an apparently healthy population of women to take a treatment for a considerable period of time with the aim of preventing potential illnesses later in life. Compliance with HRT, although often good in the short term, is usually poor in the longer term. This is due to a combination of factors including adverse side-effects, fears over breast cancer and poor understanding of long-term HRT benefits from sustained use. Almost 40% of women advised to start HRT for bone density preservation had discontinued treatment within eight months of starting in one study, mainly because of adverse side-effects (see Table 6.20).

Table 6.20 Common side-effects of hormone replacement therapy

Estrogenic	Progestogenic
Breast tenderness/enlargement	Breast tenderness
Edema/bloating	Bloating
Headache	Headache
Nausea	Acne/seborrhea
Leg cramps	PMS symptoms
Vaginal discharge	Depression
Eye irritation	Dysmenorrhea
Breakthrough bleeding	Libido changes
	Insomnia
	Lethargy
	Scalp hair loss
	Hirsutism

PMS, premenstrual syndrome

Table 6.21 Routes of administration of hormone replacement therapy

Route	Preparation
Oral	Tablets
Transdermal	Patches
	Gels
Vaginal	Creams/gels
	Rings
	Pessaries
Subcutaneous	Implants
Intramuscular	Injection
Intranasal	Spray

Choice of therapies

Changing the dosage or route of treatment can attenuate certain of the adverse effects of HRT. Beneficial metabolic effects of HRT have been demonstrated for the oral and transdermal routes of administration, and both routes have been shown to be effective in relieving postmenopausal symptoms, as well as beneficial in preventing postmenopausal bone loss. It is important to emphasize this to women about to embark on long-term treatment, since better compliance will usually follow if the patient is allowed free choice of her therapy or is encouraged to try alternatives if the first dosage or route of treatment is unacceptable. HRT can be given via various routes (Table 6.21), which should allow individualization of therapy.

The basic hormonal substances used in HRT preparations are only few, but various routes of administration and dose permutations have led to more than 50 systemic and topical preparations currently being licenced for use in the UK. Commonly used estrogens are estradiol, CEE, estrone and estriol. Commonly used progestogens are dydrogesterone, levonorgestrel, medroxyprogesterone and norethisterone.

Traditionally, oral routes of administration have been most widely used for HRT. Long-term compliance with oral regimens has been poor, but with the advent of better and less irritant patches, both the oral and the transdermal routes are becoming increasingly popular and might be expected to encourage compliance, especially with the introduction of seven-day patches. In a recent study approximately 90% of women did not miss a single application of a matrix-type seven-day patch (FemSeven) over a period of 18 months. In addition, the newer matrix patches seem to represent an improved option over reservoir patches in terms of skin reactions and improved adhesion.

Knowledge of the pharmacokinetics of oral and transdermal estrogen is useful in predicting the possible effects of treatment via these two routes. Oral estrogens are subject to extensive first-pass metabolism before metabolically active compounds can act systemically. Thus, larger doses are required than with transdermal delivery systems, which avoid this first-pass effect. Oral estrogen administration is associated with alterations in bile composition which leads to a greater degree of gastrointestinal disturbance and increased risk of gallstone disease. The transdermal route is preferred in cases of chronic liver disease, liver transplant or history of gallstones. Oral estrogens are known to exert a beneficial effect on serum lipoprotein levels via their extensive hepatic metabolism, but recent studies have also shown that transdermal estrogens exert beneficial effect, albeit to a lesser extent, on cholesterol but to a greater extent on triglyceride values. Transdermal delivery systems tend to lead to a more stable serum

Table 6.22 Mean estradiol blood levels with various hormone replacement therapy preparations

Preparation	Dose	Level (pmol/l)
CEE	1.25 mg	110–125
Oral estradiol	1.0 mg	110–130
	2.0 mg	200–225
Estradiol patches	50 µg/24 h	125–150
	100 µg/24 h	250–350
Estrodiol gel (Oestrogel)	1.5 mg	225–250
	3.0 mg	350–400
Estradiol gel (Sandrena)	1.0 mg	300–400
Vaginal ring (Menoring)	50 µg/24 h	150

CEE, conjugared equine estrogens

estradiol level than with orally administered estrogen, and may be more appropriate, for example, in women using enzyme-inducing drugs or who smoke. Cigarette smoking is thought to reduce estradiol bioavailability via its effect on hepatic metabolism, but since transdermal estradiol avoids first-pass liver metabolism, it may be less affected than oral estrogen by the effects of cigarette use. There may be a theoretically lower risk of VTE with transdermally administered estrogen replacement. Although firm evidence is lacking, it is possible that patients suffering from conditions such as hypertriglyceridemia, fibrocystic breast disease or migraine may be better suited to transdermal therapy. In addition, transdermal therapy is a good alternative for women who prefer not to take daily oral medication or who absorb medications poorly because of gastrointestinal malabsorption syndromes (e.g., post-surgery, Crohn's disease, etc.). Often, women ask for a blood estrogen level estimation. Generally, if the symptoms are controlled, the blood level is likely to be adequate and no estrogen blood level is necessary. Estradiol blood level measurement is sometimes indicated in anxious patients, if there are difficulties in symptom control or when monitoring estrogen treatment for osteoporosis. An estradiol level in excess of 200 pmol/l is considered satisfactory. Typical plasma estradiol levels reported in pharmacokinetic studies are given in Table 6.22.

Oral estrogens, including CEE, give wise to plasma estrone levels. Estrone is 3–10 times less potent than estradiol and is not measured by most laboratories. In pharmacokinetic studies, usually only estradiol is studied and there are limited data on estrone. Estrone measurement is unnecessary when prescribing estradiol.

Patient profiling

Patients' understanding of the menopause and the benefits of HRT use on their future health could be improved with dedicated well women clinics, leaflets and posters in the surgery. The initial assessment should include age of menopause and type (i.e., natural or surgical), presence of menopausal symptoms and their severity, risk factors for future heart disease, osteoporosis or other diseases potentially modified by HRT, and contraindications to HRT. Selection of the most appropriate dose and route of administration can then be made using the initial assessment according to the woman's individual needs or co-morbid illness. This should improve patients' satisfaction with care, allowing early intervention and tailoring of therapy, and should improve the take-up and continued use of HRT. Review of patients should occur at least every six months to ensure compliance, and more frequent follow-up visits may be necessary if unacceptable side-effects occur. Treatment can be altered as necessary if there are significant side-effects, or lack of symptom control. Early and easy access to a specialized menopause clinic should be offered to any patient with resistant symptoms or side-effects, or pre-existent medical problems that may complicate postmenopausal hormone therapy. Breast and pelvic examinations should be performed if clinically indicated and routine mammography (every three years) should continue while HRT is being used.

Women about to undergo hysterectomy with or without oophorectomy should be counseled regarding the benefits and risks of HRT by the gynecologist prior to surgery. A decision regarding the use of HRT should be possible well in advance of the operation. Good communication between the surgeon and the general practitioner should avoid delays or interruptions in treatment. Counseling about

Table 6.23 Causes for premature ovarian failure

Idiopathic
Turner's syndrome
Autoimmune
Chemotherapy
Familial
Pelvic surgery
Pelvic irradiation
Galactosemia
46XY gonadal dysgenesis

the benefits and possible risks of HRT is particularly important in young women with surgically induced menopause, since these women are at especially high risk of future problems, as discussed above.

PREMATURE OVARIAN FAILURE

Premature ovarian failure (POF) is the cessation of normal reproductive function before the age of 40 and is seen in about 1% of women. Patients may present clinically with either primary or secondary amenorrhea, or with menstrual irregularity or with hot flashes, sweats, fatigue, irritability or depression. The diagnosis is confirmed by the finding of elevated gonadotropin levels, measured on three separate occasions, one to two months apart. The causes of POF are numerous (Table 6.23), but they all converge in a common pathway of accelerated follicular loss. Most cases are idiopathic (about 55–60%), the second in prevalence being Turner's syndrome (20–25%).

Investigations beyond those confirming POF need not be extensive. Chromosomal analysis is necessary for women with primary amenorrhea if there are features suggestive of a chromosomal abnormality. The presence of the Y chromosome increases the risk of a germ cell tumor. The connection between POF and autoimmune disease should be considered and periodic screening for subclinical thyroid disease, adrenal insufficiency, pernicious anemia and antinuclear antibodies is often practiced. Ovarian biopsy does not add information which leads to change of management and is not recommended.

The young woman who is found to have POF requires a great deal of emotional support. Because POF is currently untreatable, it puts the patient at greatly increased risk of CVD and osteoporosis, and the diagnosis has major implication for sexual relationships, sex, sexuality and fertility. It is of paramount importance that patients understand the nature and prognosis of their condition, not least because it helps their acceptance of long-term hormone replacement. HRT will minimize the risk of CVD and osteoporosis, will alleviate menopausal symptoms if present, will bring sexual maturation and development of secondary sexual characteristics in infantile women and will restore and enhance sexuality. Often higher than usual doses of estrogen are necessary in these unfortunate patients. Androgen replacement should be offered to women who, in spite of adequate estrogen replacement, continue of complain of persistent fatigue, loss of determination and general well-being, and low sex drive. Androgen is best administered via subcutaneous implants, 50–100 mg every four to six months. In about a quarter of cases with POF (especially in idiopathic cases or after chemotherapy) there is spontaneous reversal of the condition and patients may start menstruating again or even become pregnant. It may be useful to monitor such patients by stopping HRT every one to two years for three months and measuring their gonadotropins. However, the fertility prognosis is generally poor and those patients desiring a family should be encouraged to think in terms of adoption or egg donation. Provisions for long-term follow-up should be in place to provide continuous support and health surveillance, and to monitor HRT.

SELECTIVE ESTROGEN RECEPTOR MODULATORS

The search for an even safer alternative to HRT has led to the evaluation of several compounds, previously referred to as 'antiestrogens'. Initially, these compounds were used for the treatment of hormonally responsive cancers, such as breast cancer. Therefore, they were termed 'antiestrogens'. One such compound is tamoxifen. However, after the realization that postmenopausal women with breast cancer treated with tamoxifen had lower cholesterol and increased spinal bone density compared with untreated controls, it became evident that the term 'antiestrogen' did not fully describe these compounds. The term selective estrogen receptor modulators (SERMs) has been suggested in order to define more precisely these substances, which are capable of binding to and activating ERs, but which have effects on target tissues that are different from those of estradiol. Newer SERMs are raloxifene, droloxifene and toremifene. The estrogen agonist/antagonist properties of SERMs are not fully understood and are difficult to explain. One major mechanism appears to be a change in the conformation of the ER; another mechanism lies in differences in recruitment of co-activators and co-repressors; and a third mechanism is by activation/deactivation of different classes of ERs. For example, raloxifene seems to activate predominantly ERβ and only to a lesser extend ERα which accounts for the lack of stimulation of the breast or uterus. For a more detailed discussion of ERs the reader is referred to Chapter 2. The fundamental concept behind SERMs is to try and maintain the beneficial effects of HRT while avoiding its drawbacks, especially with regard to endometrial stimulation, breast cancer and prothrombotic changes.

The one SERM that has been particularly well studied in radomized clinical trials in menopausal women and that is licensed for use is raloxifene. It, like estrogen, reduces bone remodeling in estrogen-deficient early postmenopausal women and induces a positive calcium balance shift. At 60 mg/day, raloxifene leads to an increase of bone mineral density in the spine and the hip and a reduction in vertebral fracture rates. Raloxifene decreases LDL, Lp(a) and fibrinogen, increases HDL-2, but not total HDL, and has no effect on triglycerides or PAI-1. During a median of 40 months of treating postmenopausal women for osteoporosis,

there was a 76% reduction in newly diagnosed invasive breast cancers. Raloxifene does not cause endometrial stimulation or breast tenderness, but does cause DVT at a rate similar to that of HRT. The effects of raloxifene on CHD and stroke was studied in the Multiple Outcomes of Raloxifene Evaluation (MORE) trial, a randomized controlled trial of menopausal women with osteoporosis. It recruited 7705 patients who were followed for 4 years. There was no difference in the rates of coronary events or stroke between the treatment and placebo groups. A subgroup analysis found that women with a high risk of CHD or stroke may even benefit from the treatment. Reassuringly, raloxifene does not seem to affect cognitive function. Overall raloxifene is well tolerated with discontinuation rates in clinical studies similar to placebo, but it may slightly worsen hot flashes and it can cause leg cramps in a small percentage of women. It is very likely that in future new SERMs will be developed and their indications will broaden to include relief of estrogen deficiency symptoms, prevention of breast cancer, treatment for fibroids, endometriosis, uterine cancer, etc.

NON-HORMONAL STRATEGIES FOR IMPROVEMENT OF WOMEN'S HEALTH IN THE MENOPAUSE

Bisphosphonates

Bisphosphonates are chemical analogs of pyrophosphate which bind strongly to bone to exert anti-resorptive effects which lead to improved bone density. They become incorporated at the site of bone resorption (pits) where they: (1) change physico-chemical characteristics of the bone and reduce the rate of its dissolution; (2) reduce the rate of formation of new pits; and (3) exert cytotoxic effects on osteoclasts. Bisphosphonates are poorly absorbed orally and have to be taken on an empty stomach. Three types of bisphosphonates are widely used – etidronate, alendronate and risedronate. All three increase the bone mineral density at clinically relevant site (radius, spine, neck of femur) and decrease the incidence of fractures. When taken for two years positive changes in bone density of 3–8% have been reported. Alendronate is available as a once a week dose (70 mg) which makes administration even simpler. For many women with osteoporosis, bisphosphonates may be the treatment of first choice.

Phytoestrogens

Phytoestrogens have a structure resembling estrogen and are found in plants. They have mixed estrogenic/antiestrogenic properties, the estrogenic effect being 500–1000 times less than that of estradiol. There are several different classes of phytoestrogen, but most prominent in the human diet are phenolic ones – flavones, isoflavones, lignans, coumestans. Isoflavones are the most common form of phytoestrogens and are found in a variety of fruits and vegetables but are particularly abundant in leguminous plants and especially soy. The phytoestrogens found in foods are 'precursors' because they undergo complex transformation in the gut, being metabolized by the bacteria, and then in the body. The end result is appearance in the blood of the active constituents: daidzein, genistein and equol. The daily consumption of isoflavones in Japan and other Asian communities has been estimated at 25–45 mg/day, but it is much less in the typical 'Western' diet. Observational studies and laboratory experiments have linked high consumption of phytoestrogens with low incidence of CVD, osteoporosis and cancer of the breast, colon, prostate and uterus. Those observational data have various epidemiologic deficiencies and cannot prove a cause and effect relationship.

The only rigorously tested association is between intake of phytoestrogen and hot flashes. Randomized controlled trials have shown that phytoestrogens (in the form of soy flour) have modest activity in curtailing the severity of hot flashes. It seems, therefore, sensible that menopausal women should be encouraged to increase their intake of phytoestrogens, which not only may relieve their hot flashes, but may also have wider health benefits. Daily intake of 20–60 g of soy protein or soy flour has been most widely used in clinical studies, but this may not be easily achievable in day-to-day life. Phytoestrogen tablets and isolates are less effective. According to two studies ipriflavone (synthetic isoflavone) prevents bone loss in postmenopausal women with low bone mass. Other studies investigating the effects of phytoestrogens on lipid metabolism and the cardiovascular system demonstrated a decrease in cholesterol and improved vascular function. No good data is available on phytoestrogens and cancer.

Herbs

Medicinal herbs are crude drugs of plant origin used for treatment of diseases, often of a chronic nature, or to promote good health. Herbs for treatment of menopausal symptoms have been available long before the discovery of HRT. A number of such herbs are currently widely advertised by the health food industry, which claims improvements in hot flashes, mood and general well-being. Some examples are ginkgo (*Ginkgo biloba*), gingseng (*Panax gingseng*), St John's wort (*Hypericum perforatum*) and valerian (*Valeriana officinalis*). Of these, only St John's wort has been properly researched and has been shown to be effective in mild to moderate depression. Its side-effects include gastrointestinal symptoms, allergic reactions, dizziness, confusion, tiredness/sedation and a dry mouth. St John's wort interacts with many medications in a way which may reduce or potentiate their efficacy and/or plasma concentration, because it reduces the cytochrome P450 enzyme system. Medications the activity of which is diminished by St John's wort are warfarin, cyclosporin, oral contraceptives, anticonvulsants and digoxin. The effect of triptans (i.e., sumatriptan) and selective serotonin reuptake inhibitors (i.e., fluoxetine) is increased, which leads to increased incidence of adverse reactions. Doctors should always ask about self-medication, including the use of herbal products. Natural progesterone creams

Table 6.24 Risk factors for cardiovascular disease (CVD)

Age
Male sex
High low-density lipoprotein cholesterol
Reduced high-density lipoprotein cholesterol
Raised blood pressure
Smoking
Diabetes
Family history of CVD
Obesity
Sedentary life-style
Homocystinemia

are not efficacious in prevention or treatment of osteoporosis. Their role in abating hot flashes is still under investigation. Indeed, the Medicines Control Agency issued advice that women using oral contraceptives should not use St John's wort because the latter might result in unwanted pregnancy.

Diet, exercise, smoking and weight control

As mentioned earlier in the chapter, coronary artery disease is the leading cause of death and cerebrovascular disease and stroke is the third most common cause of death in most developed countries. Women tend to present with less severe symptoms, but suffer higher mortality and are under-investigated in comparison with men. Many dozens of putative risk factors have been put under scrutiny over the years, but the number of proven ones is relatively small (Table 6.24).

Stopping smoking, weight reduction, taking up exercise and proper diet are far more important interventions on population levels than is treatment with HRT to decrease the incidence of CHD. During the last two decades the incidence of CHD has declined, smoking has declined and the diet of many people has improved. Sadly, the level of physical activity has declined and that of obesity has vastly increased. Women that do not smoke, have a healthy, varied diet, exercise and maintain a normal BMI are 80–90% less likely to develop CHD than the general population. So primary prevention of CHD should revolve around this premise. All women should be given comprehensive dietary advice, educated to have a diet rich in fruits and vegetables and low in saturated fat, and should be encouraged to try and maintain a cholesterol level appropriate for their age. Evidence from cohort studies suggests that eating more fruit and vegetables reduces the risk of heart attack and stroke. Eating fish, especially oily ones, is also beneficial. Dietary modifications in older age are often difficult to achieve and sustain even in patients with significant obesity and hypercholesterolemia. Therefore education about diet should start early in life. A diet rich in calcium and vitamin D helps with skeletal integrity after the menopause. This is more important for citizens of northern countries such as the UK, where the cutaneous synthesis of vitamin D is suboptimal because of insufficient exposure to sunlight. An additional 1.0 g of elementary calcium has been recommended after the menopause but the value of such supplementation is questionable with a well-balanced diet. The recommended daily intake of vitamin D is 400 IU (10 mg), but 700 IU of vitamin D may be advisable for citizens of northern countries who have little sunlight exposure. Sources of vitamin D are oily fish, egg yolk, liver, butter, fortified milk and margarine. Sources of calcium are listed in Table 6.25. Physical activity (moderate level of activity daily for 30 min) leads to 30–50% reduction in relative risk of CVD compared with people who are sedentary, after adjusting for other risk factors. The bone protection benefit of weight-bearing exercise is well established in the hip and it should be encouraged in postmenopausal women. Physical activity may bring a number of other health benefits (Table 6.26), and should be encouraged. The link between obesity and cancer mortality can be considered well established. Recent data suggest that obesity is responsible for 20% of all cancer deaths in the USA.

Smoking is strongly related to overall mortality and especially increases the risk of CHD and stroke. The risk of CHD and stroke

Table 6.25 Calcium content of some foods*

Food	Calcium
Cheddar cheese	674
Milk	120
Yogurt	180
Cottage cheese	60
Butter	24
Canned sardines in oil	550
Haddock	55
Bread	75
Spinach	93
Broccoli	100
Green beans	86
Baked beans	45
Carrots	37
Peas	26
Orange	51
Almonds	234

*All entries expressed as mg per 100 g portion

Table 6.26 Some conditions for which exercise is beneficial

Cardiovascular disease
Diabetes
Fracture risk
Poor postural balance
Colorectal cancer
Breast cancer

declines rapidly in both men and women two to four years after stopping smoking. Hypertension is undoubtedly a major risk factor for CHD and stroke. In people with essential hypertension, some modest reduction of the blood pressure and the risk of complications can be achieved with non-pharmacologic measures such as exercise, a low fat/high fruit and vegetable diet, reduced alcohol consumption, salt restriction and weight loss. There is no good evidence about the effect of magnesium supplements. The role of antioxidants has not been well defined. One systemic review of epidemiologic studies found a consistent association between increased dietary or supplementary intake of vitamin E and lower cardiovascular risk and a less consistent association for β-carotene and vitamin C. A randomized controlled trial using 500 mg of vitamin C and 400 IU of vitamin E ($n = 108$)

or placebo ($n = 105$) did not find any effect on coronary artery stenosis after a mean of 2.8 years of follow-up. The Heart Protection Study, a double-blind placebo-controlled trial of 20 536 subjects aged between 40 and 80 years, randomized patients to 600 mg vitamin E, 250 mg vitamin C and 20 mg β-carotene daily or placebo. After a follow-up of 5 years no differences were noted between the groups with regard to fatal and non-fatal MI, stroke, cancer or overall mortality. Both these studies were published in 2002. This is in concordance with earlier studies, some of them big ($n > 29\ 000$) and long (follow-up > 12 years), not showing beneficial effects of supplements. The fact that HRT and vitamins and antioxidants are not as effective as previously thought does not leave our patients short of options. As mentioned earlier lifestyle interventions are excellent for both primary and secondary prevention of CVD. For secondary prevention of CHD and stroke, treatment of hypertension, diabetes, high cholesterol and other risk factors with diuretics, β-blockers, ACE inhibitors, calcium-channel blockers, statins, antiplatelet agents, etc. is safe, well established and proven intervention that decrease both morbidity and mortality.

SUMMARY

The physiologic changes in women around and after the menopause are complex and not completely understood. Some of these changes are due to the aging process and some undoubtedly have a hormonal basis. The normal menopause occurs because of aging (not the other way around) and for some time it was widely thought that the clock can be turned back by use of HRT. This belief may have been over-optimistic, but it was not frivolous – there was a mountain of experimental and observational data to support it. Estrogen was thought to prevent CHD, improve mood, cognition, sexuality and well-being, delay the onset or change the severity of Alzheimer's disease and improve stress incontinence. This was on top of the well known effects on the bone, vasomotor symptoms and urogenital atrophy. The

Table 6.27 Absolute differences in the rates of major, potentially fatal diseases per 10 000 postmenopausal women per year from western countries using HRT based on results from randomized trials

Disease	Differences in events
Coronary heart disease	8
Stroke	8
Pulmonary embolism	8
Invasive breast cancer	8
Hip fracture	5
Colorectal cancer	6
Total mortality	No difference

HRT, n = 10872; placebo, n = 10 437; of those on HRT 91% were on 0.625 mg of CEE and 2.5 mg of MPA and the rest on estradiol

pharmaceutical industry responded with developing numerous estrogenic agents, regimens and routes of administration. Hormonal preparations were widely prescribed and poor compliance lamented by doctors and policy makers. With the results of a number of randomized controlled trials being published the current state of affairs is changing. The main conclusions are that: (1) the results are not immediately generalizable to all women and for all HRT preparations; (2) for many women the risks overweight the benefits; (3) women with established CHD or stroke should not take certain continuous combined HRT preparations; (4) the absolute risks of HRT are small; (5) some suspected benefits are now established, e.g., on incidence of hip fracture and bowel cancer; (6) women should not start HRT with the sole aim of preventing CHD; (7) in normal women with mild or no vasomotor symptoms continuous combined HRT (0.625 mg of CEE and 2.5 mg of MPA per day) does not improve quality of life in terms of sleep, sexual or cognitive function or body pains; (8) hot flashes are not deadly, but can be very disabling and short-term use (2-3 years) of HRT in healthy women is safe and effective treatment to relief this symptom. Table 6.27 gives a summary of risks and benefits of HRT based on most published controlled trials.

REFERENCES

(1) Herrington DM, Reboussin DM, Brosnihan KB, *et al.* Effects of estrogen replacement on the progression of coronary artery atherosclerosis. *N Engl J Med* 2000;343:522–9

(2) Waters DD, Alderman EL, Hsia J, *et al.* Effects of hormone replacement therapy and antioxidant vitamin supplements on coronary atherosclerosis in postmenopausal women. *J Am Med Assoc* 2002;288:2432–40

(3) Clarke SC, Kelleher J, Lloyd-Jones H, *et al.* A study of hormone replacemtn therapy in postmenopausal women with ischemic heart disease: the Papworth HRT Atherosclerosis Study. *Br J Obstet Gynecol* 2002;109: 1056–62

(4) Hulley S, Grady D, Bush T, *et al.* Randomized trial of estrogen plus progestin for secondary prevention of coronary heart disease in postmenopausal women. *J Am Med Assoc* 1998; 280:605–13

(5) Grady D, Herrington D, Brittner V, *et al.* Cardiovascular disease outcomes during 6.8 years of hormonal therapy. Heart and Estrogen/Progestin Replacement Therapy Follow-up (HERSII). *J Am Med Assoc* 2002;208: 49–57

(6) The ESPRIT team. Oestrogen therapy for prevention of reinfarction in postmenopausal women: a randomised placebo controlled trial. *Lancet* 2002;360:2001–8

(7) Rossouw JE, Anderson GL, Prentice RL, *et al.* Risks and benefits of estrogen plus progestin in healthy postmenopausal women: principal results from the Women's Health Initiative randomized controlled trial. *J Am Med Assoc* 2002; 288:321–33

(8) Viscoli CM, Brass LM, Kerman WN, *et al.* A clinical trial of estrogen replacement therapy after ischemic stroke. *N Engl J Med* 2001; 345: 1243–9

(9) Wassertheil-Smoller S, Hendrix S, Limacher M, *et al.* Effect of estrogen plus progestin on stroke in postmenopausal women. The women's Health Initiative: a randomized trial. *J Am Med Assoc* 2003;289:2673–84

Sexually transmitted infections and common genital tract infections

7

Alison Stirland, Chris Wilkinson and Nikolai Manassiev

INTRODUCTION

Sexually transmitted infections (STIs) and their sequelae such as infertility and chronic pelvic pain cause significant physical and psychologic morbidity. The diagnosis of an STI affects well-being, self-confidence and personal relationships.

Many of those infected are unaware that they have an STI, as symptoms are often absent or non-specific. STIs are frequently multiple, so the presence of, say, warts or gonorrhea should lead the practitioner to consider other infections, such as chlamydia. Many factors can lead to the individual to delay or avoid seeking treatment, including embarrassment, fears of stigma, concerns about confidentiality, lack of awareness of STIs and ignorance or denial of the risk of infection. Prompt diagnosis and treatment of STIs is, however, important for both personal and public health as it reduces that chance of the individual developing complications and transmitting the infection(s) to others. The presence of some STIs (gonorrhea,

herpes, syphilis, chancroid) leads to disruption of the surface barriers of the body (skin, mucosa) and facilitates HIV transmission. Thus, detecting and treating STIs also reduces the incidence of HIV.

The transmission of STIs can be lowered by changes in sexual behavior (abstinence, mutual monogamy and safer sex practices) and infection control programs (screening, early diagnosis, treatment of those infected, contact tracing and immunisation).

The burden of STIs is notoriously difficult to estimate. It varies according to the population studied, i.e., sex, age, race, occupation, education, rural, urban or inner city area are all important factors. The rates seen at genitourinary medicine (GUM) clinics are higher than those seen at general practice. Many infection episodes are asymptomatic so any reported rate is likely to underestimate the real situation. Some recent epidemiologic data are depicted in Table 7.1.

Table 7.1 New cases of STIs seen at genitourinary medicine clinics (England 2001) and new sexually acquired HIV infections (UK 2001)

Sexually transmitted infection	Cases (n)		Rate per 100 000 individuals aged 15–44 per year	
	Male	*Female*	*Male*	*Female*
Uncomplicated gonorrhea	15 476	6 642	153	65
Uncomplicated chlamydia	29 166	38 248	288	373
Herpes simplex (first attack)	6 492	10 558	64	103
Genital warts (first attack)	32 636	29 568	323	288
Infectious HIV	598	98	6	0.95

Data derived from New Cases seen at Genitourinary Medicine Clinics: England 2001. Public Health Laboratory Service (PHLS) Communicable Disease Report, 2001 and the Population Estimates Unit, Office of National Statistics, UK. HIV, human immunodeficiency disease

GENERAL CONSIDERATIONS

Managing sexually transmitted infections in primary care

In the UK, GUM clinics have the best facilities for diagnosing and managing STIs. Attending a specialist clinic, however, may not always be practical or acceptable. Basic management of common STIs and other genital infections lends itself to protocols and so readily falls within the scope of appropriately trained doctors and nurses working in general practice and family planning. The ability to manage STIs in primary care is rapidly increasing with recent advances in diagnosis and single-dose therapy. Nucleic acid amplification techniques (NAATs), polymerase chain reaction (PCR) and ligase chain reaction (LCR) are increasingly available. They are more sensitive than many antigen and culture tests and are less dependent on rapid transport to the laboratory than cultures. Effective single-dose antibiotic therapy is now available for some STIs (gonorrhea and chlamydia) and for other non-sexually transmitted genital infections (candidiasis and bacterial vaginosis (BV)).

The diagnosis of an STI can have a major impact on the personal life and health of a patient. While making a positive diagnosis is important, so is reliably excluding STIs. It is therefore vital that quality standards are applied to the whole process of managing STIs (Table 7.2). To ensure that their patients can access the full range of services, it is important that individual practices have links with local GUM clinics and microbiology laboratories.

When to refer to genitourinary medicine services

Patients should be referred to a GUM clinic when a specialist service or an expert opinion is required. On-site microscopy at GUM clinics enables presumptive diagnoses of gonorrhea and syphilis and definitive diagnoses of candidiasis, trichomonas and BV to be made at the first visit. These clinics have facilities

Table 7.2 Management of sexually transmitted infections

History and examination
Sexual history
Gynecologic history
Genital, pelvic and abdominal examination
General physical examination including mouth and
 skin, if indicated

Investigations/diagnosis
Decide
 which diagnostic test should be taken and when?
 which site(s) to sample
Optimize quality of specimens
 good sampling
 appropriate transport media
 correct storage and rapid transport of specimens to
  laboratory

Treatment
Ensure correct treatment is given, taking into account
 local antibiotic resistance patterns and possibility of
 pregnancy
Consider epidemiologic treatment
Partner notification (contact tracing)
Counseling (emotional and sexual difficulties)

Patient information (verbal and written)
Confidentiality of service
Limitations of tests – which diseases have been tested
 for
Sequelae of infection
Effect of disease and its treatment on pregnancy and
 contraception
Transmission to partners (safer sex, asymptomatic
 shedding of herpes and wart virus)
Advise abstinence until partner(s) fully treated
Health promotion (strategies to reduce the risk of
 re-infection)

Follow-up
Carry out test of cure if indicated
Enquire about patient compliance (medication and
 abstinence)
Ascertain if partner(s) treated

Administration
Practice confidentiality policy
Liaison with local laboratory and genitourinary medicine
 service
Regular review of practice and audit

to inoculate culture media for gonorrhea, herpes and trichomonas directly, optimizing sensitivity. Therefore referral to a GUM clinic is recommended for patients with genital ulceration, suspected gonorrhea and recurrent vaginal discharge. Patients with conditions

Table 7.3 Establishing the sexual history of a patient

Question	Relevance
Number of partners	
Regular partner(s)	Establishes the risk of STIs and
Non-regular partner(s) in the last 3 months	facilitates partner notification (if an STI is detected)
For each partner	
Partner's gender and the nature of the sexual contact (i.e., receptive or insertive, vaginal, oral or anal intercourse)	Establishes the risk and nature of a potential STI and indicates which site to test
Length of relationship/date of last sexual contact	Together with incubation periods, provides a guide when to perform tests
Condom use	Establishes the risk of STIs and provides an education and counseling opportunity
Partner's symptoms or diagnosis	Risk of STI, choice of test*
Overseas contact	Consider tropical diseases and resistance to gonorrhea therapy

*For example, if partner has symptoms suggesting gonorrhea, practitioner should consider testing multiple sites, repeating negative tests or offering epidemiologic treatment. STI, sexually transmitted infection

requiring specialist tests or treatment such as tropical diseases and syphilis should also be referred. Patients with warts should be offered referral to a GUM clinic for treatment, especially if they are pregnant or do not wish to use podophylotoxin at home.

Referral to or liaison with the health advisor at the GUM clinic should be considered for partner notification (contact tracing). Health advisors also provide counseling and health education. Finally, patients may prefer the relative anonymity and confidentiality of a GUM clinic if they feel uncomfortable consulting their usual practitioner about an STI or sexual difficulty.

Sexual history

Patients are unlikely to object to questions about their sexual relationships and previous STIs if they appreciate their relevance, especially if they perceive themselves to be at risk of infection. Seeking permission to ask personal questions, reassuring about confidentiality and only seeking information that will affect management, increases the acceptability of taking a sexual history (Table 7.3).

The use of gender-neutral terms such as 'partner' is helpful, as the women may be lesbian or bisexual. Some infections such as trichomonas can be spread between women, especially if sex toys are used, and some lesbians may be at risk of STIs from heterosexual contact in the past. Lesbians do not require contraception and so are less likely to attend family planning and well-women sessions. They should be offered STI testing and cervical cytology examination as appropriate. It is recognized that the comfort level and skills to talk about sex may vary between practitioners and their relationships with patients.

Women who report sexual assault should be offered referral for both forensic (if they have not already reported the incident to the police) and clinical examination. If the woman chooses to have a forensic examination, it should be performed before the clinical examination. Assessment centers, known as 'rape suites', exist in some areas and are usually located in hospitals or police stations. They specialize in the forensic assessment of both male and female victims of sexual assault. According to the woman's history, knowledge of the assailant and nature of the

Table 7.4 Testing for sexually transmitted infections (STIs): indications

On demand
Identified risk
Clinical features of STI
Under 25 years of age
New partner in previous 6 months
More than one partner in previous 12 months
High-risk partner (e.g., symptomatic or has an STI or multiple partners)
Recent history of an STI (consider re-infection)
Before clinical procedures
  termination of pregnancy
  IUD insertion
  other intrauterine procedures
    (laparoscopy and dye injection, hysteroscopy, hysterosalpingogram, endometrial biopsy, dilation and curettage)

IUD, intrauterine device

Table 7.5 Clinical features of genital infections including sexually transmitted infections*

Vaginal or urethral discharge
Vulval or pubic pruritis
Genital malodor
Vulval or peri-anal pain
Lesions (ulcers or lumps)
Dysuria
  internal (urethral or bladder pain)
  external (urine in contact with inflamed vulva)
Dyspareunia (superficial or deep)
Abdominal or pelvic pain and tenderness
Abnormal bleeding
  intermenstrual
  postcoital
  contact bleeding from cervix
Inflammation of vulva, vagina, cervix, peri-anal area and anal canal

Signs of pelvic inflammatory disease
Cardinal
  cervical excitation
  uterine or adnexal tenderness (usually bilateral)
Additional signs (may be present but are not essential for diagnosis)
    pyrexia (oral temperature > 38.3°C/> 101°F)
    adnexal mass
    lower abdominal tenderness
    peritonism
    cervical or vaginal mucopurulent discharge

*Note: the absence of symptoms or signs does not exclude a sexually transmitted infection

assault, clinicians should offer emergency contraception, hepatitis B vaccination and testing or prophylactic treatment for STIs and HIV. Counseling and referral to support organizations should also be offered.

Who to test for sexually transmitted infections

Symptoms and signs of genital infection are not specific and may be absent. Therefore women should be tested on request, if at risk (Table 7.4), or if they have clinical features of STIs (Table 7.5). Recommendations on screening await the outcome of pilot studies conducted by the Department of Health in the UK.

A woman may request STI testing for many reasons. She may be concerned about being infected by a specific partner, planning a pregnancy or seeking a check-up before starting a new relationship or discontinuing condoms. Awareness of the incubation periods of diseases is important in timing tests for STIs and in interpreting results. If a patient presents for testing during the likely incubation period, infection cannot be excluded. In these circumstances, it may be advisable to defer or repeat testing according to the risk of infection and the likelihood of her returning for follow-up. For example, if a woman presents a week after having unprotected intercourse with a new partner it may be possible to detect gonorrhea but too soon for a chlamydia test to be reliable. However, it may still be useful to test for chlamydia as she may have a pre-existing infection, and, if negative, to repeat the test after the incubation period.

It is important to explain to the patient which diseases are (and which are not) being tested for. Although a clinical diagnosis can be made from the lesions of warts or herpes, it is impossible to say, with routine tests, that a patient is not carrying herpes simplex or wart virus. The patient should also be informed of the limitations of testing, as both false-positive and false-negative results can occur. An awareness of the positive and negative predictive values of tests, such as chlamydia antigen detection, can be useful in interpreting the results as the predictive values depend on the population prevalence. The local laboratory can provide information on the accuracy of their diagnostic tests.

MAKING A DIAGNOSIS

Examination and testing of the genital area

Specimens for STI tests are taken during examination of the genital tract. In order to optimize the quality of the samples, it is suggested that the tests are taken according to the manufacturer's instructions and in the sequence set out below.

Inspect the vulval, pubic and peri-anal areas first, then pass a speculum into the vagina. If there are lesions at the introitus that would make this painful, such as herpetic ulcers, consideration should be given to deferring further examination. A high vaginal swab for *Trichomonas vaginalis*, candidiasis and BV is taken from the vaginal walls and posterior fornix and used to test for pH and sent for microscopy, culture and sensitivity (MC&S) analysis. If indicated, a cervical smear should be taken for cytology at this stage. The ectocervix should then be wiped to remove any vaginal discharge. An endocervical swab, to be sent for MC&S analysis, is then taken for gonorrhea testing. An endocervical or urinary chlamydia test should also be taken, depending on which test is offered by the local laboratory. If a cervical test is to be taken for chlamydia it is important to sample endocervical cells (as chlamydia is an intracellular organism) by rotating the swab against the wall of the endocervix (Table 7.6). The diagnosis of chlamydia and gonorrhea can be improved if urethral swabs are taken in addition to cervical samples. Urethral tests require samples to be taken with a narrow swab or loop and can be uncomfortable and are unacceptable to many women. Testing the rectum and pharynx for gonorrhea should be considered if the partner has urethral gonorrhea and anal or oral (fellatio) intercourse has

Table 7.6 Basic testing for sexually transmitted infections (triple swabs)

Organism/condition tested for	Test performed
High vaginal swab	
Candida and trichomonas	Microscopy, culture and sensitivity
BV	Microscopy as above
Endocervical swab	
Gonorrhea	Microscopy, culture and sensitivity
Endocervical swab or urine*	
Chlamydia	Use most sensitive test available locally, these may include: EIA, LCR, PCR, DIF, culture
Vaginal discharge	
BV and trichomonas	pH, using narrow range pH paper
BV	Amine test

*Depends on test used; EIA, enzyme immunoassay; LCR, ligase chain reaction; PCR, polymerase chain reaction; DIF, direct immunofluorescence; BV, bacterial vaginosis

occurred. A bimanual pelvic examination should be performed to detect signs of pelvic inflammatory disease (PID), uterine or ovarian pathology. This is especially important if gonorrhea or chlamydia is suspected or there is a history of pelvic or low abdominal pain or dyspareunia. A general physical examination including the mouth and skin may reveal signs of parasitic infection, syphilis, HIV and complications of STIs. Testing for other sexually transmissible infections such as syphilis, HIV, hepatitis B and C should be considered.

pH and amine testing

In community settings a preliminary assessment of vaginal discharge may be made by noting the character of the discharge, the presence of inflammation and by testing the pH; some also advocate amine testing (Table 7.7). Vaginal discharge may not be typical and these tests are not sufficiently specific to

Table 7.7 Features helpful in the preliminary assessment of vaginal discharge

Organism/ condition	Classic description of discharge	Inflammation of vagina	pH	Amine test
Bacterial vaginosis	Grey, thin, homogenous	Absent	> 4.5	Positive
Trichomonas vaginalis	Yellow/green, thin, frothy	Present	> 4.5	Positive
Candida Spp.	White, curdy	Present	< 4.5	Negative

provide a definitive diagnosis but may be useful especially where microscopy is not available. A sample of vaginal secretion should be placed on pH paper such as Whatmans narrow range pH paper. Care should be taken to avoid sampling cervical mucus or lubricant placed on the speculum, which would artificially raise the pH. pH testing is also unreliable in the presence of semen, menstrual fluid, vaginal treatments such as spermicides, douches and some systemic drugs. The pH is normal (< 4.5) in candidiasis but > 4.5 in BV and trichomoniasis.

The amine test is performed by adding a drop of 10% potassium hydroxide to a sample of vaginal discharge on a glass slide. Amines are released which can be detected by their characteristic odor. The amine test is positive in BV or trichomoniasis (because of the accompanying overgrowth of anaerobes) and weakly positive with menstrual blood or semen. Potassium hydroxide is corrosive and should be handled and stored with care.

Transport and storage of specimens

If specimens cannot be plated for culture at the time of collection, appropriate transport media should be used. A charcoal-based medium, for example, is often recommended for gonorrhea culture. High vaginal and endocervical swabs for bacterial culture should be kept at room temperature. Urine specimens for bacterial culture and swabs for viral and chlamydia culture usually require refrigeration and the temperature needs to be maintained until the specimen reaches the laboratory.

Individual practices should check the manufacturer's instructions and seek advice from their local laboratory. If a significant delay in the transport of cultures to the laboratory is likely for a patient with suspected gonorrhea, immediate referral to a GUM clinic should be considered.

TREATMENT OF SEXUALLY TRANSMITTED INFECTIONS

Suitable treatment should be given after considering patient compliance and the possibility of allergy, drug interaction, method of contraception, pregnancy, lactation and antimicrobial resistance. Antimicrobial treatment may be given when an STI is suspected from the patient's history, after a tentative diagnosis has been made or after it has been confirmed. Decisions on the timing of therapy should be made according to the risk of infection, the availability of diagnostic testing and the likelihood of the patient returning for results and abstaining from sexual intercourse. Treatment on epidemiologic grounds can be given to a patient whose partner is known to be infected. For example, a woman who has been having unprotected intercourse with a man with gonorrhea may be offered treatment before a diagnosis has been made. Investigations to confirm or exclude the diagnosis and exclude other STIs should still be performed, but treatment is given without waiting for the results.

All patients should be advised to abstain from sexual intercourse until they and their partner(s) have completed the treatment and tested negative (if a test of cure has been performed). Information should be offered about the disease and its treatment and how to reduce the risk of further infection and transmission. A follow-up visit is recommended to ascertain if the condition has resolved, check patient compliance and find out whether partner(s) have been notified. It is also an opportunity to provide further information and counseling for emotional and sexual difficulties. At follow-up, a test of cure should be performed for gonorrhea and trichomonas infection in all women and for chlamydia in women treated with erythromycin. As even intelligent patients may find it difficult to absorb all the information due to embarrassment and anxiety, written information should be offered.

Partner notification (contact tracing)

Partner notification involves informing sexual contacts that they have been exposed to STIs. The purpose is to prevent treated patients from being re-infected, detect their partner(s) undiagnosed infection(s) and to reduce STIs in the community. The rationale is that every patient has caught an STI from one or more partners and may subsequently infect others. Infected partners (contacts) may not appreciate their risk of infection and/or be asymptomatic.

The benefits of partner notification are greatest for the bacterial STIs because they can be cured and the risk of sequelae can be reduced by prompt treatment. Partners with incurable viral STIs, such as genital herpes and HIV, can be given information about the infection and advice on strategies to reduce the risk of transmission. All can be offered testing for other STIs including HIV and advice about safer sex.

The patient is usually advised to ask her/his partner to attend a clinic for testing and treatment. It is useful to provide a contact slip or note with the diagnosis for the contact to give to their healthcare worker. In order to maintain confidentiality, no information about the patient or contact(s) should be given to anyone

else without their permission. In practice, it is preferable to seek permission to disclose the name of the infection(s) that the patient acquired so that an adequate explanation of the disease, tests and any necessary treatment can be given to the contact. Naming the infection prevents the partner assuming that it is HIV. A patient may be reluctant to inform her partner(s) that they have an STI but be willing to provide information to enable a health professional, such as a GUM clinic health advisor, to do so. It is common practice to contact all partners with whom the patient had sexual contact in the 3 months prior to diagnosis.

BACTERIAL CERVICITIS AND PELVIC INFLAMMATORY DISEASE

Gonorrhea

Gonorrhea is an STI caused by the bacterium *Neisseria gonorrhoeae*, a Gram-negative intracellular diplococcus. Although gonorrhea is not common in many parts of the UK, sporadic outbreaks occur and the infection is endemic in many inner cities. In 2001 the rate of gonorrhea in female GUM clinic attendees in England was 65/100 000. There is wide regional variation with rates being highest in Greater London (over 165/100 000). There has been a recent increase in infection rates, especially amongst women under 20 years of age.

The incubation period of *N. gonorrhoeae* is 3 to 5 days. The common sites affected are the endocervix, urethra, pharynx and rectum, which may be infected by anal intercourse or contamination with vaginal discharge. Gonococcal conjunctivitis can also occur. Gonorrhea is asymptomatic in up to 50% of women with genital infection and in up to 90% of those with pharyngeal infection. Knowledge of local gonorrhea rates and a high index of suspicion are required to optimize opportunities for testing.

When present, symptoms include abnormal vaginal discharge, dysuria and symptoms of upper genital tract infection such as low abdominal pain, dyspareunia and intermenstrual bleeding. Gonorrhea can also present as a Bartholin's abscess. There may be no abnormal clinical signs, but there may be mucopurulent endocervical discharge, contact bleeding and signs of PID. Coexistent urethral infection is common but discharge is rarely apparent in women.

The main complication is PID; disseminated infection causing arthritis and skin lesions is rare. Very occasionally pericarditis, endocarditis, hepatitis and meningitis are seen. Vertical transmission can lead to opthalmia neonatorum, which is a notifiable disease.

Diagnosis

If gonorrhea is suspected, specimens should be taken from the urethra and rectum in addition to the endocervix. The oropharynx should also be tested if fellatio has occurred.

Microscopy demonstrates the typical appearance of Gram-negative intracellular diplococci within polymorphonucleocytes. Microscopy of an endocervical sample gives a presumptive diagnosis in 20–50% of women but should not be used for pharyngeal specimens. Culture provides definitive diagnosis and antibiotic sensitivities. If gonorrhea is strongly suspected but the test results are negative, some advocate re-testing prior to treatment.

Treatment

Treatment for gonorrhea should be guided by local antibiotic resistance patterns, which are monitored by microbiology laboratories or GUM clinics. Resistance to penicillins, tetracyclines and quinolones occurs, especially in cases imported from locations overseas such as South East Asia. Penicillins should only be used as a first-line treatment if the incidence of resistance is known to be low. Pharyngeal gonorrhea responds poorly to penicillins (Table 7.8). As many women with gonorrhea are also infected with chlamydia, it is common practice to treat with a combination of antibiotics effective against both organisms. After treatment further cultures should be performed to detect treatment failure or re-infection.

Table 7.8 Single-dose treatment regimens for gonorrhea

a) Women who are not pregnant or lactating

	Drug (dose)
Uncomplicated genital gonorrhea	
Oral	Ampicillin (2 g) with probenecid (1 g)
	Ciprofloxacin (500 mg)
	Ofloxacin (400 mg)
	Levofloxacin (250 mg)
Alternative regimen for uncomplicated genital gonorrhea imported from South East Asia	
IM	Ceftriaxone (250 mg)
	Cefotaxime (500 mg)
	Spectinomycin (2 g)
Pharyngeal gonorrhea	
Oral	Ciprofloxacin (500 mg)
	Ofloxacin (400 mg)
IM	Ceftriaxone (250 mg)

b) Pregnant and lactating women*

	Drug (dose)
Uncomplicated genital gonorrhea	
Oral	Ampicillin (2 g) with probenecid (1 g)
IM	Ceftriaxone (250 mg)
	Cefotaxime (500 mg)
	Spectinomycin (2 g)

*Quinolones and tetracyclines are contraindicated in pregnant and lactating women; IM, intramuscular

Chlamydia trachomatis

Chlamydia trachomatis serotypes D to K are obligate intracellular bacteria that cause a genital infection with a similar clinical presentation to gonococcal infection. Chlamydia is much more prevalent than gonorrhea and is less confined to inner city areas. Longstanding asymptomatic genital infection is not uncommon: up to 75% of infected people have no symptoms. Establishing a sexual history is therefore important to identify women who are at risk of chlamydial infection.

The rate of chlamydia is highest in sexually active teenagers. High prevalences have also been reported in women seeking termination of pregnancy (Table 7.9) and following intrauterine device (IUD) insertion for emergency contraception. In 2001 the reported rate of chlamydia in England was 373/100 000, with higher rates being observed

Table 7.9 Prevalence of chlamydial infection in women (19–44 years) reported from various clinical settings in the UK, 1997–2001

Population	Median prevalence (%)	Range (%)
General population	1.5	1–2
General practice	4.5	1–12
Gynecology clinics	4.8	3–6
Family planning clinics	5.1	3–7
Women seeking abortions	8.0	7–12
GUM clinics	16.4	7–29

GUM, genitourinary medicine. Data derived from Chlamydia Trachomatis. Summary and Conclusions of CMO Expert Advisory Group. London: Department of Health

in Greater London and considerably lower ones in East Anglia and the South West of England.

The incubation period of *Chlamydia trachomatis* is approximately 2 weeks. The main sites of infection are the urethra and cervix, although the pharynx and rectum may also be involved. When present, symptoms include vaginal discharge, mild dysuria, intermenstrual and postcoital bleeding and lower abdominal pain with dyspareunia. Contact bleeding from the cervix may be noted on examination. Pharyngeal and rectal infections are usually asymptomatic, although rectal pain and anal discharge may be reported. Rarely, Chlamydia causes adult conjunctivitis, perihepatitis and sexually acquired reactive arthritis (SARA). When transmitted vertically, the neonate may develop opthalmia or pneumonia. Chlamydia is responsible for the majority of cases of PID. Chlamydia causing only minimal symptoms and signs of PID can cause chronic pelvic pain, tubal damage and subfertility. However, the risk of infertility should not be overemphasized, so that the woman does not discontinue her method of contraception. Chlamydial infection has also been estimated to account for 40% of ectopic pregnancies.

Diagnosis

A number of speciments can be used to test for chlamydia. Trained medical professionals can take swabs from the cervix and urethra. The cervix needs to be cleaned of excess mucus or discharge before swabbing. The cervical swab should be inserted 1–2 cm into the cervix past the squamocolumnar junction and turned several times in order to exfoliate columnar cells. A second swab is taken from the urethra. The urethral swab is inserted 1 cm into the urethra and rotated 1–2 times. Both swabs are usually transported together.

First voided morning urine is an excellent specimen for nucleic acid amplification assay. The first 10–20 ml of the morning urine contain epithelial cells from the urethra and may contain chlamydia. Urine specimens have the advantage of being simple and non-invasive, but specimens need to be maintained at low temperatures during transportation to the laboratory. Vaginal swabs obtained by the patients themselves have also been shown to be good specimens for chlamydia testing.

NAATs such as LCR and PCR are more sensitive than culture tests or enzyme immunoassays (EIA or enzyme-linked immunosorbent assay (ELISA)) and, if available, are the diagnostic methods of choice. LCR and PCR may be useful as screening tests as they can often be carried out on urine specimens, avoiding the need for a vaginal examination. The full potential of these tests is still being evaluated. Direct immunofluorescence (DIF) and culture tests are expensive and unsuitable for analyzing a larger number of specimens. Culture tests are required in forensic cases, such as rape, in view of their high specificity.

Treatment

Uncomplicated chlamydial infection in non-pregnant women should be treated with doxycycline 100 mg orally twice daily for 7 days or azithromycin 1 g orally as a single dose. Women who are pregnant, lactating or who do not tolerate these drugs may be treated with erythromycin stearate 500 mg orally twice daily

Table 7.10 Findings supporting a diagnosis of pelvic inflammatory disease

Oral temperature > 38.3°C (> 101°F)
Cervical and/or vaginal mucopurulent discharge
Presence of WBC on microscopy of vaginal secretions
Elevated ESR
Elevated CRP
Laboratory diagnosis of *N. gonorrhoeae* or *C. trachomatis*

WBC, white blood cells; ESR, erythrocyte sedimentation rate; CRP, C-reactive protein

for 14 days. Erythromycin leads to a slightly lower cure rate than doxycyline, so patients treated in this way should be re-tested three weeks after completing therapy.

Screening

In the UK, there is no routine screening for chlamydia. Patients are tested for chlamydia only when it is clinically indicated or to perform opportunistic screening in high-risk groups. Table 7.4 lists indications when testing for STIs (including chlamydia) should be instituted.

Pelvic inflammatory disease

PID is an ascending pelvic infection, which may produce a combination of endometritis, salpingitis, oophoritis and parametritis. It may be complicated by tubo-ovarian abscess, pelvic peritonitis and peri-hepatitis. It is usually related to cervical infection with *N. gonorrhoeae* or *C. trachomatis*. The latter is responsible for most cases, although the bacteria may coexist. Anaerobic bacteria associated with BV (bacteroides, anaerobic cocci) may also be involved in the pathophysiology of PID. Other microorganisms found in patients with PID include *E. coli*, *Mycoplasma hominis* and ureaplasma.

PID is more common in women under 35 years old and in those with multiple partners or an STI. It is rare in pregnancy, before menarche or after menopause. Hormonal and barrier (condoms, diaphragm) methods of contraception appear to be protective. PID is not always due to an STI and can occur after a gynecologic procedure in the absence of either chlamydia or gonorrhea. The risk of PID after termination of pregnancy is approximately 5–15% and less than 1% following IUD insertion. These rates are highest if there is a pre-existing cervical STI. The risk of pelvic infection with an IUD *in situ* is only raised above the background risk for 20 days after insertion. It has been demonstrated that the rate of postabortal PID can be approximately halved when prophylactic antibiotics are used at the time of termination of pregnancy. The Royal College of Obstetricians and Gynaecologists' Guidelines recommend that selected women are tested for STIs and/or given prophylaxis before an intrauterine procedure (see page 59 for reducing the risk of PID in women having an IUD fitted).

Diagnosis

Women may be asymptomatic, but it is more common that PID presents with lower abdominal pain, deep dyspareunia, vaginal discharge and intermenstrual bleeding. The diagnosis of PID is usually made on clinical findings, as the gold standard, laparoscopy, is rarely used. The only findings on examination required to make a diagnosis of PID are cervical, uterine or adnexal excitation (cervical motion tenderness) and adnexal tenderness. In addition, the patient may also be pyrexial and/or have abdominal tenderness, signs of peritonism or a pelvic mass. Right upper abdominal pain suggests the presence of peri-hepatitis, a rare condition associated with both chlamydial and gonococcal PID, known as the Fitz–Hugh–Curtis syndrome. Other complications of PID are tubo-ovarian abscess, pyosalpinx and hydrosalpinx. A raised white blood cell count, C-reactive protein or erythrocyte sedimentation rate supports the clinical diagnosis of PID, retrospectively. Because of the need to carry out effective contact tracing, testing for STIs is important. A pregnancy test may be required to exclude ectopic pregnancy. Other differential diagnoses to consider include acute appendicitis, torted or ruptured ovarian cyst and endometriosis. Additional criteria supporting a diagnosis of PID are listed in Table 7.10.

Treatment

Early treatment of PID reduces the risk of developing long-term sequelae such as ectopic pregnancy, infertility, chronic pelvic pain and dyspareunia. The risk of developing subfertility is approximately 9% after one episode of PID and approximately doubles with each subsequent episode. The risk of ectopic pregnancy for women with a history of PID is 10%. Therefore, there should be a low threshold for treatment. As PID is polymicrobial, combination antibiotic therapy is required to cover gonorrhea, chlamydia and anaerobic infection.

Treatment depends upon local patterns of antibiotic resistance but usually consists of oral doxycycline 100 mg twice daily for 14 days plus oral metronidazole 400 mg twice daily for 14 days and ciprofloxacin 500 mg stat. Hospital admission and parenteral treatment is indicated for more severe clinical disease, particularly in the presence of HIV infection (Table 7.11). One in-patient regimen is cefoxitin 2.0 g IV every 6 h plus doxycycline 100 mg orally or IV every 12 h. Analgesia may be required. When PID is diagnosed in a patient with an IUD, it is advised to leave the device in place unless the condition has not improved 48 h after starting treatment.

Patients should be advised to avoid intercourse until they, and their partner(s), have completed treatment and follow-up. Clear verbal and written information should be provided. Pelvic examination should be performed at follow-up visits, 2 days and 2 weeks after commencing treatment.

VAGINAL INFECTIONS

Vaginal discharge is a common complaint in sexually active women. Normal discharge in premenopausal women is non-irritant,

Table 7.11 Indications for hospital admission

Diagnostic uncertainty
Clinical failure with oral therapy
Presence of a tubo-ovarian abscess
Inability to tolerate oral therapy
Immunodeficiency

non-offensive, not blood-stained and has a pH of 3.5–4.5. Normal vaginal flora includes *Corinebacterium, Bacteroides, Peptostreptococcus, Mobiluincus, Gardnerella, Mycoplasma* and *Candida* spp. The acidic pH, which serves a protective function, is maintained by lactobacilli, which produce lactic acid. There are no glands in the vagina. Vaginal discharge originates predominantly from vaginal desquamation, bacteria and secretions from the cervix and upper genital tract. It may be, therefore, a presentation of upper genital tract disease including infection and, rarely, malignancy.

The important symptoms in women with abnormal vaginal discharge are pruritis, odor, intermenstrual bleeding (including postcoital bleeding) and abdominal pain. On examination, in addition to the color and nature of the discharge itself, the presence of vulvitis, vaginitis and cervicitis should be noted.

Whilst the commonest causes of vaginal discharge, BV and candidiasis, are not sexually transmitted, the same symptoms can be caused by other conditions and the possibility of an STI should be considered. Foreign bodies like retained tampons usually result in vaginal discharge. Atrophic vaginitis and allergic reactions to bubble baths, douches and other cleansing or perfumed agents can cause soreness and itching.

If an STI is suspected, appropriate tests should be performed or the patient referred to a GUM clinic. It is common practice to treat empirically if an STI is *not* suspected and many patients self-medicate with, e.g., antifungal therapy. However, it is important that women should be examined and investigated if symptoms persist.

Table 7.12 Treatment of bacterial vaginosis

	Regimen
Non-pregnant women	
Metronidazole orally	400 mg twice daily for 7 days
Metronidazole orally	2 g as a single dose
Clindamycin 2% vaginal cream*	One applicator full each night for 7 days
Pregnant women (or suspected pregnancy)	
Metronidazole orally	400 mg twice daily for 7 days

*Clindamycin cream may weaken latex condoms, diaphragms and cervical caps and is contraindicated in pregnancy

Bacterial vaginosis

BV, also referred to as anaerobic vaginosis, is a cause of vaginal discharge but is non-sexually transmitted. It is common with a prevalence of up to 20%. BV is characterized by an altered vaginal bacterial flora with a preponderance of anaerobic bacteria, such as *Mobiluncus spp.*, *Gardnerella vaginalis*, *Bacteroides spp.* and *Mycoplasma spp.*, and an absence of lacto-bacilli. The etiology of BV is poorly under-stood. Although it is related to sexual activity, a sexually transmitted pathogen has not been identified and BV can occur in women who are not sexually active. There is an association with vaginal douching and the use of IUDs.

BV may predispose women to postopera-tive pelvic infection, endometritis after birth or termination of pregnancy, chorioamnioni-tis, second trimester loss, premature birth and rupture of membranes. It is also believed to play a role in the pathogenesis of PID.

Vaginal discharge and fishy odor may occur but approximately half of all women with BV have no symptoms. As BV does not cause inflammation of the vagina and vulva, a com-plaint of soreness or pruritis should lead to consideration of coexistent conditions. The clinical findings are malodor and thin, grey, homogenous vaginal discharge.

Diagnosis

The diagnosis of BV is made if three of the following four criteria are present: (1) thin white/grey discharge; (2) vaginal pH > 4.5; (3) positive amine test; and (4) clue cells detected on microscopy of a wet mount or gram stain. Clue cells are vaginal epithelial cells coated in Gram-variable bacilli that have a characteristic appearance on microscopy. Where immediate microscopy is not available, the history, clinical findings and a raised vagi-nal pH suffice for a presumptive diagnosis. Setting up a culture for *Gardnerella vaginalis* is not helpful in the diagnosis of BV.

Treatment

Women with a diagnosis of BV should be offered treatment (Table 7.12), even if they do not report symptoms as some may not regard their discharge as abnormal or are too embarrassed to mention symptoms such as odor. Treatment is advised for women with BV who are pregnant, especially if they have symptoms, a history of late miscarriage or premature labor. The value of routinely screening asymptomatic women in pregnancy has not yet been demonstrated.

BV may resolve spontaneously but recur-rences are common and frequently noticed after menstruation or intercourse. Treating the male partner(s) does not prevent recur-rence. Follow-up tests are not performed if the patient is no longer symptomatic, except in pregnant women with a history of late miscar-riage or premature labor who should be re-tested after 1 month.

Vulvo-vaginal candidiasis

Candidiasis is caused by the yeast *Candida*. Over 90% of cases are due to the *C. albicans* species, most of the remainder being due to *C. glabrata*. About 60–70% of women experi-ence at least one episode of candidiasis in their lifetime. Such factors as reduced immu-nity, steroid therapy and undiagnosed dia-betes are occasionally involved in recurrent infection. It is not sexually transmitted, although some male partners develop mild, pruritic balanitis soon after intercourse, which usually resolves within 24 h.

Table 7.13 Treatment of vaginal candidiasis

	Regimen	Notes
First-line therapy		
Clotrimazole (vaginal pessary)	500 mg single dose nocté or 200 mg nocté for three nights or 100 mg nocté for six nights	Effect on latex contraceptives is unknown
Fluconazole (oral tablet)	150 mg single dose	Contraindicated in pregnancy
Second-line therapy		
Miconazole (vaginal ovule)	1.2 g single dose nocté	Damages latex contraceptives
Econazole (vaginal pessary)	150 mg single dose nocté or 150 mg nocté for three nights	Damages latex contraceptives
Nystatin (vaginal cream or pessary)	100 000 units nocté for 14 nights	Cream, but not the pessary, damages latex contraceptives

Diagnosis

The most notable symptoms are vulval pruritis and a white vaginal discharge. Soreness and superficial dysuria and dyspareunia may also be present due to inflammation and fissuring of the vulva. The clinical findings may vary from very mild to severe vulvo-vaginitis with a typical white curdy discharge. Vulval erythema usually has a marked edge and adjacent satellite lesions may be present.

In GUM clinics, the diagnosis of vulvo-vaginal candidiasis is made by detecting yeast and pseudohyphae on microscopy of vaginal discharge on a gram stain or wet slide prepared with 10% potassium hydroxide. The pH of vaginal discharge is usually less than 4.5 unless BV and/or trichomonas is also present. In community settings a presumptive diagnosis can be made by clinical findings and a normal pH. Culture confirms the diagnosis and the causative species.

Treatment

Ten to twenty per cent of women of child-bearing age and 30–40% of pregnant women may have *Candidiasis* asymptomatically and do not require treatment. The mainstay of treatment of candidiasis is with azoles, many being available without prescription (Table 7.13). Topical therapy such as clotrimazole 1% cream is useful for vulvitis but should not be used alone to treat vaginal candidiasis. After treatment no specific follow-up is required. Male partners do not require treatment. Balanitis usually resolves if unprotected vaginal intercourse is avoided until the vaginal infection is treated.

Patients with recurrent infection should be examined and tested to confirm the diagnosis of candidiasis and exclude other infections. Diabetes and immunodeficiency caused by conditions such as HIV infection and corticosteroid therapy should be considered when candidiasis recurs frequently, although these are uncommon causes of candidiasis in the general population. Patients can be advised to avoid products such as bubble baths and vaginal deodorants and tight underwear made of synthetic fabric, if these appear to exacerbate the condition. Prophylactic drug regimens for recurrent infection are empirical and include clotrimazole 500 mg pessaries one every 1 or 2 weeks. Women who notice symptoms of candidiasis occurring premenstrually can be treated 2 days prior to the anticipated onset of symptoms. Women prone to candidiasis during antibiotic therapy can also be offered prophylaxis. In women with a history of recurrent candidiasis, treatment of the male partner should be considered.

Trichomoniasis

The flagellated protozoan *Trichomonas vaginalis* (commonly known as TV) causes trichomoniasis, which is almost always sexually transmitted. It is uncommon, compared with BV and candidiasis, and is asymptomatic in up to half of cases. The incubation period of *T. vaginalis* is 1 to 3 weeks. It affects the vagina and urethra and has no long-term complications. It is a cause of non-specific urethritis (NSU) in men. The diagnosis of trichomoniasis should alert the clinician to test for presence of other STIs.

Diagnosis

Clinical features range from no symptoms or signs to a severe vulvo-vaginitis with profuse vaginal discharge and abdominal discomfort. There is usually marked erythema of the vaginal epithelium and the classic 'strawberry cervix' is occasionally seen. The discharge may be malodorous, blood-stained and frothy and yellow/green in color.

The diagnosis, suspected by clinical features and a vaginal pH above 4.5, is made by culture or microscopy analysis of a wet mount from a high vaginal swab. As it has a low specificity, trichomoniasis suspected on cervical cytology should be confirmed by culture or microscopy analysis. Both trichomoniasis and BV cause a raised vaginal pH, but the former can usually be distinguished from the latter by the presence of vaginal inflammation.

Treatment

Oral metronidazole is recommended as either 2 g in a single dose or 400 mg twice a day for

Table 7.14 Causes of genital ulceration

Herpes simplex
Syphilis
Chancroid
Lymphogranuloma venereum
Granuloma inguinale
Trauma
Malignancy
Anogenital amoebiasis
Behcet's syndrome
Crohn's disease

5 days. The single high-dose regimen should be avoided in pregnancy. Male partners should be examined and tested for trichomoniasis and other STIs. As culture or microscopy analysis for trichomoniasis is insensitive in men, partners should be treated for it, even if the organism is not detected.

A test of cure should be performed in women. Successful treatment is dependent upon patient compliance and the simultaneous treatment of her partner(s). If resistance occurs and re-infection has been excluded, advice on further treatment should be obtained from a microbiologist or GUM physician.

GENITAL ULCERS

Genital ulceration is common. Whilst the vast majority of cases are due to the herpes simplex virus, it is important to differentiate between those that are due to trauma, infection or cancer (Table 7.14). Traumatic ulcers are usually due to chronic rubbing or localized scratching. Ulcers caused by infectious diseases usually clear without treatment. Malignant ulcers, which may appear similar, should be suspected by their failure to heal. A diagnosis should be sought in all cases of genital ulceration.

Genital herpes simplex virus

Genital herpes, a common STI, is usually caused by herpes simplex virus (HSV)-type 2 but an increasing proportion of new cases are due to type 1 (HSV-1). In 1998 the estimated rate of first-time genital herpes nationally was 103/100 000 women aged 16–44 (Table 7.1). In London the rate was considerably higher at almost double this number. A UK study published in 2000 found that the prevalence of HSV-1 antibodies was 24.5% in a random sample of children under 15 years of age (almost certainly representing oro-labial HSV infection) and 54% in women aged 25–30 years of age. HSV-2 antibodies were detected in the sera of 3.3% of men and 5.1% of women over the age of 16 years. Higher prevalences of 10.4% and 12.4% were reported in London from antenatal patients and blood donors, respectively. A representative national sample of non-institutionalized US population aged > 12 found HSV-2 prevalence of 26% and 18% in females and males, respectively. Prevalence in African-Americans was more than double that of the Caucasian sample. Higher prevalence for HSV-2 is found in homosexual men, GUM clinic patients, HIV sero-positive persons and commercial sex workers. Symptoms of genital herpes due to HSV-1 tend to be milder and recurrences are less frequent. HSV is transmitted during genital and oro-genital (including oro-anal) contact. Both types, most commonly HSV-1, can also cause oro-labial and ocular herpes. Important factors in the spread of herpes are under-diagnosis due to absent or atypical symptoms and asymptomatic shedding. The incubation period is approximately 3 to 10 days.

Terminology

Primary genital infection is the term used when initial infection with HSV-1 or -2 occurs. This is usually associated with a clinical episode. Common sites of viral entry are the vulva, peri-anal area, vagina and cervix. There is cross-reactivity between antibodies to HSV-1 and -2, so primary infection with HSV-2 tends to be mild or asymptomatic in individuals with previous exposure to HSV-1 and vice versa.

The first episode is the first recognizable clinical episode of genital herpes. This can occur a long time after the primary genital infection. Thus, it is not possible to be dogmatic about when the actual infection was acquired.

Recurrent episodes and asymptomatic shedding

HSV exhibits latency in the sensory root ganglion of the site of entry. Reactivation can give rise to both recurrent symptomatic episodes and asymptomatic shedding. A person with herpes can infect others when the virus reactivates as they shed the virus from the genital area or mouth. It is not possible clinically to detect when a person is shedding virus. The majority (about 70%) of cases of genital herpes are transmitted by viral shedding when the patient is asymptomatic because people with herpes tend to avoid intercourse when they are aware that they have a recurrence. Discordant couples who avoid intercourse during identified recurrences have an estimated transmission rate of 10% per annum.

Clinical features

Primary genital herpes The features of primary genital herpes vary widely and unrecognized infection is common. Primary herpes may be asymptomatic or cause local symptoms at the site of viral entry and/or systemic illness. The typical description of primary genital herpes is of a flu-like syndrome with fever, malaise and myalgia. Associated autonomic neuropathy may lead to urinary retention, constipation and aseptic meningitis. Rarer complications are skin, joint, liver or lung involvement. Three to four days after the onset of the systemic illness, multiple vesicles develop at the site of infection. The blisters can become small, sometimes pinpoint ulcers, or coalesce to form a large lesion resembling a syphilitic chancre. The lesions are very painful and cause severe dysuria and vaginal, urethral or rectal discharge according to their location. There is associated bilateral tender inguinal lymphadenopathy and edema. Complete healing can take 2–3 weeks.

Recurrent genital herpes Individuals with recurrent genital herpes may experience a prodrome, typically neuralgic type pain, tingling, itching and hyperasthesia at a localized site where a lesion is to develop. The lesions are few in number and tend to recur at the same site with each outbreak. Recurrences are said to be precipitated by ultraviolet light, febrile illness, menstruation and stress, although the role of these factors is debated. Recurrences are common in the first year, especially in men and those with a prolonged first episode, but become less severe and less frequent with time.

Pregnancy and genital herpes

In comparison to genital herpes, neonatal herpes is very rare but the morbidity and mortality are high. Neonatal herpes occurs in approximately 1 in 50 000 neonates and the majority of affected babies are born to women with no history of genital herpes.

Neonatal herpes is transmitted during delivery and post-natally when babies are kissed by people with oro-labial infection or handled by those with herpetic whitlow. The risk of neonatal herpes is highest if the woman has primary herpes during her pregnancy, especially at the time of delivery. Pregnant women with partners who have a history of herpes should be advised how to avoid acquiring the infection during pregnancy. Pregnant women with primary herpes should be referred for specialist advice for consideration of aciclovir and, if late in pregnancy, of prophylactic aciclovir and Cesarean section.

The risk of neonatal herpes in an infant whose mother has a history of recurrent genital herpes is very low. Routine testing for viral shedding during pregnancy or delivery has not been demonstrated to be of value. If genital lesions are present at the time of labor, delivery by Cesarean section should be considered.

Herpes and immunocompromised patients

In the presence of HIV infection, herpes tends to be chronic and severe and worsens as the HIV infection progresses. Lesions are often large, their appearance is atypical and secondary infection is common. Intravenous therapy may be required and prophylaxis often given to prevent pain and systemic infection. Advice should be sought from a specialist in HIV medicine.

Diagnosis

The diagnosis of HIV infection may have considerable psychologic, sexual and social implications. Therefore, if suspected from clinical examination, the diagnosis should be confirmed by isolating the virus in tissue culture. Viral culture is best performed on vesicular fluid taken from the base of a fresh ulcer. Culture becomes less reliable when there is crusting or the lesion is dry. In one study the positive rate for culture in comparison to PCR was vesicle/pustule 90%, ulcer 70%, and crust 27%. Referral to a GUM clinic or liaison with a virology laboratory is necessary as the specimen must be taken with appropriate swabs and placed in viral transport or culture media kept at 4°C. Diagnosis is likely to improve when NAATs such as PCR become commercially available.

The interpretation of HSV serology is complex. Genital herpes can be caused by HSV-1 or -2 and serology may take up to 3 months to become positive after primary infection, the antibodies persist indefinately. Positive serology does not indicate when the infection occurred and therefore does not distinguish between HSV from a childhood cold sore and genital herpes in adulthood. Type-specific HSV serology is likely to become available in the UK soon, but its quality and role in clinical management and screening are yet to be established. The psychosocial impact of a diagnosis of asymptomatic HSV infection should also be considered. Type-specific serology may be useful in advising patients with their first episode of genital herpes, counseling asymptomatic partners of patients with genital herpes and in the diagnosis of recurrent genital ulceration.

Management

A patient presenting with genital herpes, in pain and unwell from a flu-like illness, needs good symptom relief, clear factual information and time for discussion. Follow-up visits and counseling are important, as psychologic or psychosexual complications are common. Issues that may arise include deciding how and when to tell new partners about herpes, feeling unclean and loss of sexual confidence and libido.

Treatment of primary episodes with oral antiviral agents reduces the severity of the illness and accelerates healing (Table 7.15). Therapy should be commenced in the first 5 days of an episode or when lesions are still appearing. Warm baths and oral analgesia provide symptomatic relief. Topical anesthetic agents such as lignocaine ointment are also helpful. Increasing fluid intake and urinating into the bath or shower can reduce external dysuria. If urinary retention occurs, it should be managed by suprapubic catheterization.

Recurrences are usually managed with symptomatic treatment alone, although episodic and suppressive therapy should be considered according to the frequency and severity of the episodes and the impact they have on the patient's life.

Episodic therapy is a 5-day course of antiviral medication given early in a recurrence to shorten its duration. Suppressive therapy or prophylaxis, taken on a daily basis, reduces the frequency of recurrences and viral shedding. A common regime is to start with oral aciclovir 400 mg twice daily and 'titrate' the dose according to the number of recurrences. Supportive therapy reduces the frequencies of recurrences by 70–80% in those with ≥ 6 recurrences per year. Prophylaxis is usually given for a year initially. Patients should be advised how to recognize recurrences so that they can avoid sexual contact at the earliest stage of an episode until the lesions have

Table 7.15 Five-day courses of oral antiviral therapy for herpetic episodes

Drug	Primary herpetic infection	Recurrent herpetic infection
Aciclovir	200 mg five times daily	200 mg five times daily
Valaciclovir	500 mg twice daily	500 mg twice daily
Famciclovir	250 mg three times daily	125 mg twice daily

healed. If they are not sure whether their symptoms are due to a recurrence they should seek further advice. Condoms may reduce the risk of transmission from asymptomatic viral shedding at other times, although the degree of protection is uncertain. Asymptomatic shedding is more frequent in the first 12 months of acquiring HSV-2.

The diagnosis should be confirmed before commencing suppressive or episodic treatment. A GUM clinic, which may have a herpes or special problems session, can provide testing, counseling and specialist advice.

Syphilis

Syphilis is a rare but important STI that may be evident on genital examination in the early, primary and secondary stages. Syphilis is included in the differential diagnosis of many conditions as its presentation is frequently not classical. It may go unrecognized unless detected by routine testing in settings such as GUM and antenatal clinics. Syphilis is caused by the spirochete *Treponema pallidum* which has an incubation period of 9–90 days, typically 21 days. In acquired syphilis *T. pallidum* enters through the mucous membranes or skin and rapidly disseminates throughout the body. The classic presentation of primary syphilis is painless local lymphadenopathy and a single papule, which erodes to form a painless indurated ulcer or chancre. The chancre heals in 4–8 weeks in untreated patients. The secondary stage, which often develops 2–8 weeks after the appearance of the chancre, is characterized by systemic symptoms such as fever and weight loss, rashes,

Table 7.16 Tropical causes of genital ulceration

Infection	Organism	Features
Chancroid	*Hemophilus ducreyi*	Painful ulcers and suppuration of the inguinal lymph nodes
Lymphogranuloma venereum	*Chlamydia trachomatis*	Vesides and ulcers which may be painless, followed by suppurative lymphadenopathy with skin sinuses and discharge; constitutional symptoms
Granuloma inguinale	*Calymmatobacterium granulomatis*	Painless beefy-red nodules and ulcers; secondary infection common; leads to gross soft-tissue destruction; no regional lymphadenopathy

generalized painless lymphadenopathy and multi-system involvement including hepatosplenomegaly. Hypertrophic papules called condyloma lata occur in moist areas and are extremely infectious. Snail track ulcers may be observed in the mouth.

Early syphilis (up to 2 years, including primary, secondary and early latent[1]) is highly infectious after which infectivity gradually declines. Late syphilis (late latent[2], tertiary and quaternary) has serious long-term neurologic, skeletal and cardiologic consequences in 30% of those who are not treated. Sequelae include dementia, sensory deficit, skeletal deformity and aortitis, which can lead to aortic regurgitation and aneurysm. Congenital syphilis is now very rare, but is preventable with effective screening and treatment.

The diagnosis is made by fluorescent techniques or dark-ground microscopy of serum from a lesion, or more commonly by serology. Serological results should be interpreted by an experienced clinician who can exclude the possibility of previous treated infection, false positives and disease caused by other treponemes such as yaws. Early disease is easily treated providing compliance is good but serology often remains positive for life. Cases of suspected syphilis should be referred to GUM clinics for diagnosis, treatment and partner notification.

Tropical diseases

Chancroid, granuloma inguinale (Donovanosis) and lymphogranuloma venereum cause genital ulceration with associated lymphatic involvement. Basic information about them is shown in Table 7.16. They are common in many parts of the tropics and are occasionally seen in the UK in patients returning from overseas. If suspected, referral to a department of tropical medicine or GUM clinic for diagnosis and management is recommended.

VIRAL INFECTIONS AND INFESTATIONS OF THE SKIN

Genital warts and human papillomavirus infection

Genital warts are tumors caused by the human papillomavirus (HPV). There are over 90 subtypes of HPV, about half of these cause diseases in man. Genital HPV is usually sexually transmitted and is the commonest of these infections with over 30 HPV subtypes implicated, notably type 6 and 11. Genital HPV has a prevalence rate of 20–46% depending on the clinical setting and country. Incidence figures for England are given in Table 7.1. Vertical transmission during delivery occurs, but complications of this are rare. Young

---

[1]Early latent disease is asymptomatic disease without evidence of tertiary or quaternary disease where the time from the original infection is known to be less than 2 years.

[2]Late latent is asymptomatic disease without evidence of tertiary or quaternary disease where the time from the original infection is greater than 2 years.

women usually become infected with HPV within a few years of becoming sexually active. Multiple concurrent and sequential infections with various (including oncogenic) types of HPV are common. Most such infections are with the low-risk subtypes (6 and 11) that are cleared, and by 12 months 70% of these women are no longer infected. Persistent infection is present in about 10% of women after 5 years, and half of these women will progress to develop precancerous lesions or cervical cancer if screening is not performed routinely.

The incubation period for genital warts is typically 3 weeks to 6 months, although longer periods do occur. Subclinical infection is very common and the factors determining which HPV-infected individuals develop warts are poorly understood. Genital warts are more common in pregnancy and in association with HIV infection.

The sites most commonly infected are the vulva and peri-anal areas. Warts can also occur in the cervix, vagina, anal canal, urethral meatus and mouth. There is a wide range of clinical findings, from lesions only visible on colposcopy to confluent exophytic genital warts. Warts can be single or multiple, flat or pedunculated, and, according to their location, are firm and keratinized or soft. Symptoms may be absent or include itching, bleeding and discomfort. Emotional and psychosexual difficulties may also occur.

HPV subtypes 16, 18, 31, 33 and 35, which may not lead to clinical wart infection, are implicated in the etiology of high-grade cervical intraepithelial neoplasia and squamous cell cervical cancer. Virtually all squamous cell cervical cancers contain DNA from one of the 18 high-risk HPV subtypes known to be associated with cervical cancer. They are also associated with vaginal and vulval intraepithelial neoplasia. However, cervical cytology should not be performed more frequently than usual in women with warts unless indicated for another reason.

Diagnosis

Genital warts are diagnosed by a careful and thorough clinical examination. Biopsy and colposcopy are performed if the diagnosis is uncertain, to exclude malignancy and pre-cancer. Biopsy is also indicated for cervical lesions.

Treatment

It is increasingly recognized that the purpose of treatment for genital warts is to improve the cosmetic appearance and reduce psychologic morbidity. Treatment does not eradicate subclinical infection and its effect on the degree and duration of infectiousness is unknown. Treatment may also fail or new warts may appear during or after treatment. Warts may also regress spontaneously without treatment. In view of these factors and as many treatments are uncomfortable and inconvenient, the therapeutic options should be discussed with the patient. Some will opt to remain untreated. Patients who are distressed may benefit from counseling.

GUM clinics provide a range of treatment options and wart treatment may be available at convenient hours without an appointment. This is important, as multiple attendances are often required. Ablative methods such as cryotherapy and electrocautery are useful for keratinized lesions whilst cytotoxic methods such as podophyllin and podophylotoxin are used on soft lesions. Electrocautery, scissor excision, laser or surgical removal, trichloroacetic acid and intralesional interferon are occasionally used in specialist centers. Podophylotoxin and imiquimod (an immune-response modifier) are available for self-application and can be useful for patients with external warts if they are confident in identifying lesions, follow instructions carefully and are not at risk of pregnancy.

Progress should be assessed weekly until the warts have been eradicated. Improvement should be seen within 3 weeks and resolution is usually achieved in 6. Specialist management should be sought for patients who are immunocompromised or who have warts affecting the vagina, cervix, urethral meatus and anal canal. Sexual partners may already be infected with HPV by the time warts

Table 7.17 Recommended treatments for external genital warts

Treatment	Application
Applied by patient	
Podophillotoxin 0.5% solution	Apply twice daily for 3 days, followed by 4 days of no therapy. Treatment can be repeated up to four cycles
Imiquimod 5% cream	Apply once at night three times a week for up to 16 weeks. Wash area after 6–10 h
Administered by healthworker	
Cryotherapy	Apply with liquid or cryoprobe. Repeat every 1–2 weeks
Podophyllin resin 15% in compound benzoin tincture	Apply to each wart and allow to dry; repeat weekly as necessary
Trichloracetic acid 80–90%	Apply to each wart and allow to dry; repeat weekly as necessary
Surgical treatment	
Electrosurgery	
Curettage	
Shave and scissor excision	

become apparent. Condoms are usually recommended for 1 month after resolution. Recommended treatments for genital warts are summarized in Table 7.17.

Pregnancy and genital warts

In pregnancy genital warts may enlarge or increase in number due to altered immunity. Treatment may be offered to reduce the size and number of lesions in an attempt to reduce neonatal exposure and lower the risk of very large lesions obstructing labor. However, it may be decided to 'wait and see' until after the delivery, as many treatments for warts are contraindicated in pregnancy, lesions tend to regress post-natally and the complications (neonatal laryngeal papillomas and obstruction of labor) are rare.

A new development in the preparation of HPV infection is a vaccine against HPV type 16. Approximately 20% of all HPV infections are of this subtype, and it is present in 50% of cervical cancers and high-grade cervical intraepithelial neoplasia. The vaccine consists of empty viral capsids; it is well tolerated and generates high levels of antibodies against HPV type 16. In one controlled clinical trial of over 2300 women, none of the vaccinated patients developed a HPV type 16 infection after a median of 17.4 months of follow-up. In the placebo group, 3.8% of women developed an infection. Immunising HPV type 16-negative women may reduce their risk of cervical cancer. Vaccines against other types of HPV are being evaluated and may help to reduce the incidence of genital warts.

Molluscum contagiosum

Molluscum contagiosum is caused by a pox virus of the same name. It is spread by skin-to-skin contact. In adults, it is usually sexually transmitted, especially when it affects the groin, genital area or lower abdomen. Mollusca commonly occur in children where they affect the face, trunk and upper limbs and are not indicative of sexual activity. Lesions appear about 1–3 months after infection. They regress spontaneously after several months but can last for up to 2 years. The lesions are usually asymptomatic or associated with mild pruritis. The clinical appearance is of papules with shiny umbilicated domes 2–3 mm across. In HIV-positive individuals the lesions may be multiple, large, prone to secondary infection and often located on the face. The diagnosis is made on clinical grounds but, if required, can be confirmed by electron microscopy of material from the core of the lesion. As an alternative to waiting for spontaneous regression, the lesions may be treated by cryotherapy, curettage, expression of the core or piercing with an orange stick dipped in phenol.

Infestations

Scabies and pubic lice are frequently spread by sexual contact so testing for STIs should be considered in infested patients. As the incubation period is approximately 4 weeks for scabies and 1–4 weeks for pubic lice, sexual partners should be treated irrespective of symptoms. Permethrin should be used with caution in women who are pregnant or breastfeeding.

Scabies

Scabies is caused by the mite *Sarcoptes scabiei* that is transmitted by skin-to-skin contact. It has an incubation period of approximately 4 weeks. Clinical features include pruritis, a rash and signs of excoriation; burrows, frequently seen on the wrists, elbows and web spaces; and nodules or papules, especially on the genital area. Secondary infection can occur especially in those with HIV who may develop highly infectious, extensive, crusted lesions. If the diagnosis is unclear, mites can be observed on microscopy of material from the burrows.

Individuals and their sexual and household contacts should be treated, whether or not they have symptoms, with permethrin 5% cream or malathion 0.5% aqueous liquid. The treatment should be applied to the whole body from the neck downwards, including the hands, and left on overnight for 12 h. If it is correctly applied, a single treatment should be sufficient in the immunocompetent. Further application may cause sensitization and thus worsen symptoms. Permethrin is the preferred treatment for patients with HIV.

Crotamiton cream and antihistamines are useful for pruritis, which may persist for several weeks after treatment, especially at the site of nodules. Bedding and clothing should be washed in hot water or left unused for 3 days, by which time the mites will have died.

Phthirus pubis (pubic lice)

Phthirus pubis is spread by close bodily contact and can affect hair on the face and body in addition to the pubic area. As the louse survives less than 24 h without the human host, fomite transmission is uncommon. The disease may be asymptomatic. Clinical features include itching, a macular rash and the presence of lice (crabs) and eggs (nits).

Malathion 0.5% aqueous liquid is recommended for the treatment of pubic lice. Alternatives include phenothrin 0.2% lotion and permethrin 1% cream rinse but these are in an alcohol base, which should be avoided by asthmatics and may irritate excoriated skin and genitalia. Treatment is applied to the whole body and dry hair and left on overnight for 12 h. Treatment should be repeated after seven days to kill any newly hatched lice. Casts of eggs remaining attached to hairs after treatment can be removed with forceps or by combing, but eggs seen at the base of hairs may signify re-infection or treatment failure. Lice affecting the eyelashes can be treated with aqueous malathion (which is not licensed for this use), removed with forceps or coated with petroleum jelly twice daily for a week. Bedding and clothing used in the previous 24 h should be washed in hot water or left unused for 24 h, by which time the mites will have died.

BLOOD-BORNE SEXUALLY TRANSMISSIBLE VIRUSES

The blood-borne sexually transmissible viruses, hepatitis B and C and HIV, are transmitted vertically, by sexual contact, intravenous drug use and by treatment or accidental inoculation with blood and its products (Table 7.18).

Table 7.18 Risk factors for sexually transmissible blood-borne viruses

Sexual contact with an infected individual or with a person with risk factors whose infection status is unknown

Sexual contact with a person from a geographical area where HIV is endemic

Vertical transmission*

Intravenous drug use

Men who have sex with men

Blood transfusion or use of blood products†

---

*Vertical transmission is not proven for hepatitis C. In countries where there is a high prevalence of hepatitis B in the heterosexual community this is a common mode of transmission for hepatitis B and the diagnosis may not be made until adulthood. HIV transmitted vertically usually becomes evident early in childhood; †the risk varies between countries, it is negligible in the UK

Table 7.19 Approximate risks of HIV transmission in various settings in Europe and the USA

Female to male	1:1000 to 1:10 000
Male to female	1:1000
Receptive anal intercourse	1:30 to 1:125
Mucous membrane exposure	1:1000
Needle stick injury	1:300
HIV-infected blood in blood transfusion	1:500 000 per unit transfused

Human immunodeficiency virus

There are two types of human immunodeficiency virus, HIV-1 and HIV-2. The majority of the estimated 49 500 cases of HIV in the UK are due to HIV-1 with less than 100 cases due to HIV-2. In the UK, approximately 4400 people are diagnosed as being HIV-positive in 2001 and 36% of new infections are attributed to heterosexual intercourse. Many people who are HIV-positive (including about 50% of those acquiring the infection through heterosexual exposure) are unaware of their HIV status. Between 1986 and 2001 the number of diagnoses of HIV infection attributed to heterosexual intercourse increased from 80 to 2444 a year. The majority (over 70%) of these are acquired abroad, predominantly in Africa. The rise in the number of infected women increases the potential for vertical transmission. The majority of cases of vertical transmission are preventable if maternal infection is diagnosed prenatally or in early pregnancy with appropriate antenatal, intrapartum and neonatal care.

The major advance in the management of men and women with HIV is the development of highly active antiretroviral therapy (HAART) which delays the onset of AIDS and death in many of those treated; it is of note that deaths due to AIDS fell by two-thirds between 1995 and 1999 and has remained at the same level since.

The risk of HIV transmission from a single act of unprotected vaginal intercourse has been estimated to be approximately 1 in 1000 from a male to a female and less for female to a male (Table 7.19). The risk is higher following unprotected receptive anal intercourse. The risk of transmission from oral intercourse is thought to be very low, but has been reported. The likelihood of infection varies considerably according to the stage of disease, therapy taken by the infected person and the presence of other conditions such as STIs. The risk is increased if other STIs are present, if sexual intercourse takes place during menstruation and in women with cervical ectopy. The risk for acquiring or transmitting HIV infection is reduced in circumcised men. Condoms, when used correctly, offer good protection against HIV transmission. Condoms or latex barriers (also known as dental dams) are recommended for oral intercourse. The value of prophylactic therapy after condom failure or unprotected intercourse with an infected person is widely debated. Prophylactic therapy is not widely available and each case should be considered individually. Prophylactic treatment for needle-stick injury is more established and should be offered to those affected. Without treatment, if the needle is contaminated with HIV, the risk of infection is estimated to be approximately 3 per 1000.

Testing for the human immunodeficiency virus

Until routine antenatal screening was advised in the UK, women were less likely to be tested for HIV than gay men and, if infected, were less likely to seek medical care, take medication and to participate in clinical trials.

When HIV infection has been recognized, the patient's immune state can be monitored and, if appropriate, prophylaxis offered for the opportunistic infections caused by *Pneumocystis carinii* and cytomegalovirus (CMV). Early diagnosis in women gives the opportunity to screen more frequently for cervical dysplasia and to provide appropriate counseling and medical management of contraception, preconception and pregnancy. Cervical dysplasia is 10 times more common in HIV-positive women and is related to immunosuppression rather than HIV itself.

Women who are aware that they are infected with HIV may qualify for certain social and welfare benefits and are able to make more informed decisions about their lives. Early diagnosis means that they have longer to live with the knowledge that they are infected and the associated psychologic and social sequelae. For many women this is overridden by the benefits of an improved prognosis, choices about pregnancy and the ability to reduce the risk of transmission to others, including their children. In addition, those too frightened to have a test may become depressed and engage in risk-laden behavior and so need support.

It is important, therefore, to make HIV testing as routine and accessible as possible. Testing should be performed only with the client's informed consent with referral to specialist counselors reserved for those who are at high risk of infection or are extremely anxious. Patients should understand the meaning of a positive and negative test and the 3-month window period. The advantages and disadvantages of testing include medical benefit, stigma, social and psychologic effects, impact on relationships, work and insurance. Any service providing HIV testing must have a protocol for managing people with positive results, who may need immediate psychologic support and medical referral. This is particularly important in areas of low prevalence where facilities and expertise may be limited. Both negative and positive results should be given in person, preferably at morning clinics, when help for those with positive results can be sought. Clients who test negative may need to repeat the tests after the window period and may require advice about how to remain uninfected.

Prevention of vertical transmission of the human immunodeficiency virus

The prevalence of HIV among women giving birth in London has risen five-fold since 1988 and in 2001 it was 0.35% in London and 0.04% in the rest of the UK. In London, the prevalence of HIV in women having a termination of pregnancy is approximately two times that of women continuing with their pregnancy. Unless maternal HIV infection is diagnosed before or in pregnancy the risk of vertical transmission is approximately 20%, and possibly as high as 30% in the developing world. Additional 12–14% are infected if the mother breastfeeds the infant into the second year. In the US Center for Disease Control study ACTG 076, vertical transmission of HIV was reduced from 25.5% to 8.3% by giving zidovudine to mothers during pregnancy and labor and to the neonate. Other interventions to reduce vertical transmission are elective Cesarean section and abstaining from breastfeeding. The combined intervention of anti-retroviral drugs, elective Cesarean section at 38 weeks and no breastfeeding reduces the risk of HIV transmission to less than 2%. The options of drug therapy, Cesarean section and alternatives to breastfeeding may not be available in the developing world. A child born with HIV despite these measures can benefit from early intervention such as prophylaxis for *P. carinii* infection. Due to the transplacental passage of maternal antibodies to HIV, the status of the neonate cannot be determined until the child is approximately 18 months old; until this time the HIV status of the child is referred to as being 'indeterminate'.

Human immunodeficiency virus infection and infertility treatment

HIV infection is not in itself a contraindication to infertility treatment and each case should be considered on its merits by the general practitioner, gynecologist and patient. Patients considering a pregnancy should see a specialist, particularly if the couple are discordant. Women with HIV require information on reducing the risk of transmission to their partner and fetus. Where the male partner is HIV-positive, recent work to reduce HIV transmission by washing semen samples prior to insemination is encouraging.

Hepatitis A, B and C

All patients seeking consultation for STIs should be advised about hepatitis A, B, and C. Although uncommon, some patients may present with symptoms, signs or laboratory findings of viral hepatitis. This brief section is a reminder to the healthcare provider not to forget that hepatitis A, B and C can be sexually transmitted.

Hepatitis A

Hepatitis A is caused by the hepatitis A virus (HAV), which is transmitted via a fecal–oral route. HAV has an incubation period of about 4 weeks (range 15–50 days). It replicates in the liver and is shed in the feces. Over 80% of infected people have symptomatic infections, but in some the infection is inapparent. Like any enteric infection, hepatitis A can be sexually transmitted. Outbreaks of hepatitis A among men who have sex with men have been reported.

In a recent survey of sexual behavior in Britain, 11% of women and 12% of men reported anal sex in the past year. Inapparent fecal contamination may be present during heterosexual intercourse. Many sexual practices and inadequate personal hygiene also facilitate the fecal–oral transmission of HAV. Condoms do not prevent the transmission. Vaccination is recommended for people at risk of sexual transmission of the virus and for drug users.

Hepatitis B and C

Hepatitis B is caused by infection with the Hepatitis B virus (HBV). HBV replicates in the liver and is found in a high concentration in the blood and in lower concentrations in other body fluids: semen, vaginal secretion, and wound exudates. A person with a chronic HBV infection is potentially infective for life. Transmission of HBV can occur in heterosexual partners and in men who have sex with men.

Other risk factors for hepatitis B are essentially the same as for HIV (Table 7.16), whereas hepatitis C is much less likely to have been acquired through sexual intercourse. People identified as having HIV or hepatitis C infection or who are carriers of hepatitis B should be referred for specialist care. Those at risk of hepatitis B who are non-immune should be offered vaccination. Hepatitis B is a notifiable disease. The incubation period for hepatitis B is approximately 40–160 days while hepatitis C serology is usually positive after 3 months.

Benign breast conditions and screening for breast cancer   8

Nikolai Manassiev

INTRODUCTION

Breast disorders account for a large number of consultations. It is estimated that 30 per 1000 women consult their general practitioner about a breast problem every year. In general surgical units, breast problems can occupy some 25% of the workload. Breast disease presents as a painless lump in 35% of women, a painful lump in 33% and as diffuse or generalized pain in the breast in 18%. Nipple discharge is the presenting symptom in about 5% of patients and a smaller percentage present as breast or nipple distortion, inflammation or eczema or change in appearance in the breast or the nipple. The bedrock of diagnosis is the so-called 'triple assessment' or a combination of (1) breast examination; (2) imaging (mammography, ultrasound); and (3) biopsy or cyst aspiration. It is important to reach a diagnosis as soon as possible because women with breast symptoms are commonly afraid that they have breast cancer. It has to be emphasized that the majority of women who present with breast symptoms do not have breast cancer. About half of all women who attend breast clinics are found to have no abnormality on examination and investigation, and a further 40% have benign disease.

CLINICAL APPROACH TO BREAST DISEASE

Nomenclature of breast disease is confusing. The simplest classification is to describe what is felt when the patient is examined, i.e., a lumpy breast or a discrete lump. By separating a discrete solitary lump from the lumpy breast, women are separated into those who will need further investigation and those who require only explanation and reassurance. The discrete solitary lump can be a fibroadenoma, a cyst or a carcinoma. Other discrete solitary lumps are rare and a detailed discussion of them is beyond the scope of this review.

A lump in the breast needs to be at least 1 cm in diameter to be detected clinically. About 30% of women have lumpy breasts. The preferred term to describe lumpy breast(s) is 'benign breast change'. Terms like chronic mastitis or fibrocystic disease are meaningless and suggest that a histologic diagnosis can be established at the time of the clinical examination when it cannot. The lumpy breast may or may not be accompanied by cyclical pain associated with menstruation. Women with no discrete lumps but with lumpiness should be reassured. They should not be let to believe that they have a disease. Similarly, young women who get cyclical pain for about a week before their menses – so-called cyclical mastalgia – should also be reassured. Brownish nipple discharge, particularly from several ducts, is usually caused by duct ectasia and is a common condition but not sinister. All other cases, particularly discrete lumps at any age, should be referred to a breast specialist (Table 8.1). Difficult cases, where it is not certain whether it is a lump or lumpiness, should also be referred. Many women consult their doctors not because of symptoms but simply because of a family history of breast cancer. It is important to explain to these women that breast cancer is a common disease that makes it likely that in some families there will be a case of breast cancer. One such

Table 8.1 Patients for whom referral to a breast specialist is recommended

Discrete mass
Persistent asymmetric nodularity
Nipple discharge, especially if blood-stained, profuse or
   in a woman above 50 years of age
Nipple retraction or distortion
Severe mastalgia
Changes in the breast skin, i.e., dimpling, tethering, etc.
Relevant family history

case in a patient's family history does not necessarily point to hereditary breast cancer but that the individual may run a higher than average risk. There are special cases where an individual is strongly predisposed to breast cancer and these should be recognized and referred to a specialist unit.

BENIGN BREAST CONDITIONS

Fibroadenoma

Fibroadenoma is the most common benign breast neoplasm and accounts for about 12% of all palpable breast lumps. They are particularly frequent in women aged 15–30 years. Fibroadenomas commonly present as a painless breast lump and some 20% are multiple. Clinical breast examination reveals a firm, mobile, smooth or lobulated non-tender mass. The impression of a benign tumor is confirmed by imaging and fine-needle cytology. The natural history of a fibroadenoma is that approximately 5% grow progressively, the majority remain the same size and about 20% regress. In women under 40 years of age, small (less than 2 cm) fibroadenomas do not need to be removed. If the lump starts to grow, however, removal is indicated. Many surgeons recommend excision of any lump in women over 40 years of age.

Breast cyst(s)

Benign breast cysts are common and most frequent in the 40–50 year age group. In one study of 725 patients who died from causes other than breast cancer, microcysts (< 1 mm) were found in 37% of women and larger cysts were detected in 21%. Breast cysts are frequently multiple, often asymptomatic and are often discovered by chance by the patient. A solitary cyst is smooth and spherical. In consistency it can vary from soft to firm to hard. Usually it is not possible to demonstrate fluctuation, fluid thrill or transillumination. The clinical diagnostic feature is its smooth round shape. When subjected to triple evaluation, they exhibit specific X-ray features and fine-needle aspiration usually obtains green to bluish–black fluid. Provided that no residual lump remains after aspiration and the fluid is not blood-stained, cytology is not necessary. If there is a residual lump, it needs to be subjected to biopsy, unless cytology suggests otherwise. Recurrence of cysts is infrequent, but if the patient is known to have recurrent cysts and presents with another lump, it is generally safe to perform aspiration without a new triple evaluation. Figure 8.1 depicts an algorithm for the management of breast lumps.

Breast pain

Breast pain is the third commonest presenting symptom of breast disease. Breast pain is either cyclical, non-cyclical or does not originate from the breast. A careful history and clinical examination usually can help distinguish between these categories. Sometimes it is helpful to ask the patient to keep a pain diary so that the nature and cyclicity of the pain can be established. Cyclical pain can become continuous as it becomes more severe. If the pain is clearly cyclical and the breast examination does not reveal a discrete lump, no further investigation is needed. If the pain is of recent onset, non-cyclical and located in one breast only, investigation with imaging is necessary. If the results of the examination and the imaging are negative, the patient has to be reassured. If the imaging gives cause for concern, a biopsy is indicated.

Non-cyclical breast pain has inflammation as the underlying pathology. It is difficult to treat, but stopping smoking and a trial of non-steroidal anti-inflammatory drug may

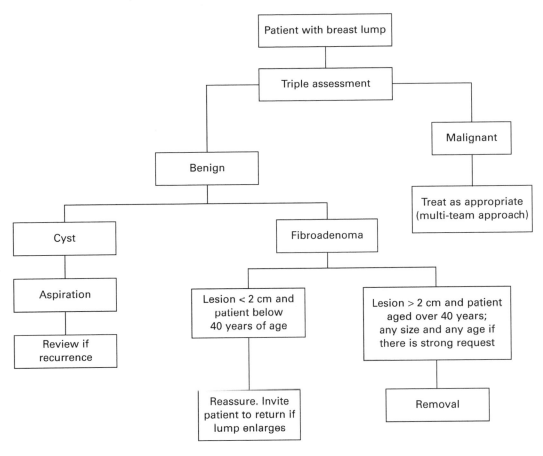

Figure 8.1   Management of breast lumps

help. If the pain is localized to a single tender spot within the breast, infiltration with local anesthetic and a corticosteroid may help. Gamolenic acid is taken by many women, but it is not usually effective.

Cyclical mastalgia

This is a condition which presents with pain lasting typically for about a week in the second half of the luteal phase. The pain is due to the effect of cyclical hormonal changes in the breast, which may increase some 10–15% in size premenstrually. Common strategies to help women with cyclical mastalgia are: properly fitting brassieres, danazol, tamoxifen and prolactin treatments, normally tried in that order. Treatment of 8–12 weeks is

recommended before assessing the result and deciding to change. Diuretic therapy and supplementation with vitamins B, B_6 and E have not been proven to be effective. Dietary manipulations (excluding coffee, tea and chocolate) can also be tried. Figure 8.2 represents a common treatment algorithm for breast pain. Until recently, gamolenic acid was commonly prescribed for breast pain. However, because of lack of effectiveness it is no longer available on the UK National Health Service (NHS).

Nipple discharge

Nipple discharge occurs in over 10% of women with benign breast disease and in 2–3% of women with cancer. In 5% of women

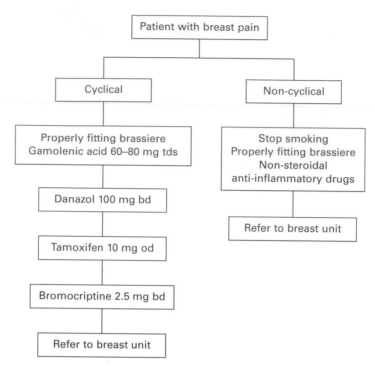

Figure 8.2 Management of breast pain. tds, three times a day; bd, twice a day; od, once a day

consulting their physician for a breast problem, spontaneous nipple discharge is the primary complaint. The discharge can be clear, milky, bloody or of green/dark color. Bilateral nipple discharge, clear or milky, in the absence of breast lump(s), excludes breast cancer and indicates systemic cause, such as a prolactinoma or medication. Unilateral clear or bloody discharge is commonly caused by duct papilloma or duct ectasia. Pressing with one finger around the periphery of the areola will reveal the culprit duct. Excision of a single duct is the recommended treatment, so intraduct carcinoma can be excluded. Some practitioners evaluate clear discharge with mammography and cytology, reserving duct excision for patients with bloody discharge. Multiduct discharge due to duct ectasia does not require treatment except for symptomatic relief. The patient should be advised to wear a properly fitting brassiere and be discouraged from aspirating the discharge or manipulating her breasts.

BREAST CANCER

Cancer is the second most common cause of death in the UK. Two in five people in Britain will have a cancer diagnosed at some time during their life and one in four will eventually die from the disease. Some recent cancer statistics are outlined in Table 8.2. Many forms of cancer are eminently treatable when discovered early but the prognosis worsens the later the cancer is diagnosed. Therefore establishing a screening program for the early detection of cancer, preferably in the preclinical stage, makes sense.

Breast cancer is the most frequently diagnosed cancer after skin cancer. In 1998 it was the most frequent cause of cancer death among British women but was overtaken by lung cancer the following year. Estimated lifetime risk of breast cancer in British women is approximately one in 11, or 9%. Because it is a cumulative risk estimate the one-in-eleven statistic, although accurate, is the most

Table 8.2 Cancer statistics for women (excluding non-melanoma)

Incidence – UK 1999		Deaths – UK 2001		Five-year survival for selected cancers (%)[*]	
Cancer	n (%)	Cancer	n (%)		
Total malignant	136 160	Total malignant	79 422	Total malignant	43
Breast	40 989 (30)	Breast	12 994	Malignant melanoma	82
Colorectal	16 811 (12)	Lung	13 038	Breast	74
Lung	14 737 (11)	Colorectal	7 630	Uterus	65
Ovary	6 800 (5)	Ovary	4 657	Cervix	61
Uterus	5 612 (4)	Pancreas	2 527	Colorectal	39
Cervix	3 202 (2.4)		3 543 (5)	Ovary	28

[*] From registration 1986–1990; data derived from Cancer Research UK May 2003
(www.cancerresearchuk.org/aboutcancer/statistics/)

Table 8.3 Risk factors for breast cancer

Factors influencing risk	Estimated relative risk
Age	Incidence strongly influenced by age
Residency in Western Europe or North America vs. Asia	4–5
Residency in urban area	1.5
Higher educational status or family income	1.5
One first-degree relative with breast cancer	2–3
Two first-degree relatives with breast cancer	4–6
Premenopausal breast cancer in mother or sister	3.0
Nulliparity or late age at first birth (> 30 vs. < 20 years)	2.0
No breastfeeding for > 6 months	1.5
Early menarche (< 12 vs. > 15 years)	1.5
Late menopause (≥ 55 vs. 40–45 years)	1.5
Biopsy-confirmed proliferative breast disease	2.0
Obesity (postmenopausal only) (≥ 200 vs. < 125 lb)	2.0
History of breast cancer in one breast	4–5
History of primary ovarian or endometrial cancer	1.5
HRT use (for 5 years after the menopause)[*]	1.35
Oral contraceptive use[*]	1.2
High alcohol intake (approx. 2 units/day)	1.4

[*] The risk disappears after 5 years of stopping the therapy; HRT, hormone replacement therapy

Table 8.4 Protective factors for breast cancer

Early first-term pregnancy
Lactation (≥ 6 months)
Physical activity
Low alcohol consumption
Diet high in fresh fruits and vegetables
Early menopause: before 45 years
Age of menarche: 20% decrease for each year that menarche is delayed after the age of 16 years

dramatic way of describing the risk. It is important to emphasize that only 25–35% of women developing breast cancer actually die from the disease – an important fact for concerned women. The estimated lifetime risk of dying from breast cancer is about 1:30–35 women. There are approximately 33 000 new cases of breast cancer a year in the UK, and the total mortality from this disease is about 13 000 a year. Rates vary, with the Far East having a much lower incidence than Western Europe and North America. Some risk factors for breast cancer are given in Table 8.3, while some protective factors are listed in Table 8.4. It should be noted that the numbers in Table 8.3 are not absolute. They tend to change as new data become available and they vary between studies. According to life tables, the potential years of life lost because of breast cancer for 1000 women is 463 as compared to 460 potential years of life lost from lung

Table 8.5 Risk of developing breast cancer in the USA stratified by age

Age interval (years)	Risk of developing breast cancer (%)
0–95	12.64
30–40	0.4
40–50	1.65
50–60	1.95
60–70	3.6
70–80	4.1
65–85	5.48

Data derived from (1) Garber JE, Smith BL. Management of the high-risk and the concerned patient. In Harris JR, *et al.*, eds. *Diseases of the Breast*. Philadelphia, PA: Lippincott, 1996:324; and (2) Feuer EJ, Wun LM. The lifetime risk of developing breast cancer. *J Natl Cancer Inst* 1993;85:892–7

Table 8.6 Risk of death from various life events per annum

Life events	Relative risk
All natural cause, age 40 years	1:850
Influenza	1:5000
Road traffic accident	1:8000
Leukemia	1:12 500
Maternal mortality	1:16 700
Playing football	1:25 000
Accident at home	1:26 000
Accident on railway	1:500 000
From one unit of blood transfused	1:5 000 000
Hit by lightning	1:10 000 000

cancer and 1535 years lost from cardiovascular disease. These calculations show that, although breast cancer is an important cause of premature death, the number of deaths it causes is approximately equivalent to that of lung cancer (a predominantly preventable disease) and vastly smaller than that of cardiovascular disease.

The background risk for breast cancer (Table 8.5) is different in different age groups. For counseling purposes, one might consider providing breast cancer risk figures for various time intervals, such as the next year, the next 10 years or a lifetime.

Appreciating the magnitude of breast cancer risk is not possible unless a comparison is made. To put this risk into context, it is necessary to give the risk of other life events. Examples are given in Table 8.6.

High-risk groups and family history

Inherited mutations in the breast cancer *BRCA1* and *BRCA2* genes predispose women to both breast and ovarian cancers, often at younger ages. *BRCA1/2*-induced cancer accounts for 5–7.5% of all breast cancer, the rest being sporadic. The pattern of inheritance in families that are carriers of *BRCA1/2* mutations is autosomal-dominant, with 50% of the offspring inheriting the mutations. For young women with high-penetrance mutation(s), the lifetime risk of developing primary breast cancer may be as high as 90%, the risk of breast cancer in the unaffected breast about 65%, and the risk of ovarian cancer may exceed 40%. Therefore, women at risk may consider preventive strategies such as tamoxifen, prophylactic mastectomy and/or prophylactic oophorectomy. Screening for *BRCA1* and *BRCA2* genes is performed in regional genetic centers, which should be able to provide referral guidelines on request.

Proper risk estimation and family tree reconstruction is possible only if at least some of the affected relatives are still alive and blood samples can be taken for genetic screening. It has been recommended that for families with *very high risk*, annual mammography and breast examination should start at an age 10 years younger than the youngest affected relative. For women with *high risk* because of the family history or simply at increased risk because of non-familial causes, annual mammography and breast examination should start 5 years before the age of the youngest affected relative, but no later than 35–40 years of age. There is no agreed definition what constitutes high risk or very high risk, but examples are: (1) *Very high risk*: two or more first-degree relatives with breast or ovarian cancer, one or more first-degree relatives with breast cancer before the age of 40 years

Table 8.7 British Association of Surgical Oncology guidelines for familial breast cancer management

High risk (refer to regional genetic center for testing)
Breast/ovarian cancer families with four or more relatives on same side affected at any age
Breast cancer in three affected relatives with average age at diagnosis under 40 years
Breast/ovarian cancer families with three affected relatives with average age at diagnosis under 60 years
Family with one relative with both breast and ovarian cancer

Moderate risk (annual mammography age 35–49; mammography every 18 months for patients above 50 years
One first-degree relative with breast cancer diagnosed at under 40 years
Two first- or second-degree relatives with breast cancer diagnosed at under 60 years
Three first- or second-degree relatives with breast cancer diagnosed at any age
Two first- or second-degree relatives with ovarian cancer diagnosed at any age
One first-degree relative with bilateral breast cancer diagnosed at under 60 years
One first-degree male relative with breast cancer at any age

Reproduced from Emery J, Murphy M, Lucassen A. Hereditary cancer – the evidence for current recommended management. *Lancet Oncol* 2000;1:9–16, with permission from Elsevier

or any first-degree relative with bilateral premenopausal breast cancer; and (2) *High risk*: any one first-degree relative, three or more second-degree relatives or any second-degree relative with breast cancer before the age of 40 years. An example of recently published guidelines from the British Association of Surgical Oncology is presented in Table 8.7. The reader should bear in mind that guidelines vary between countries and even within the same country, and do change. Guidelines should be used to justify referral pattern at all times.

Clinical breast cancer

About 85–90% of clinically discovered breast cancers present with a lump in the breast; most of the remaining 10–15% present with pain, skin or nipple retraction (5%) and discharge from the nipple (2%); pain or swelling in the axilla is also occasionally noted. Signs include a mass, tethering of the skin and reduced mobility, dimpling of the skin and nipple inversion. Skin infiltration or erosion, the classic peau d'orange and axillary or supraclavicular lymph node enlargement are signs of advanced disease. An eczematous nipple may be a sign of an underlying intraductal cancer. Occasionally, the patient may present with symptoms from secondary deposits, for example in the spine or brain. About 90% of all breast cancers originate from the epithelium lining the lactiferous ducts and ductules and are therefore typical ductal adenocarcinomas. The rest originate from the alveoli and are lobular adenocarcinomas. Intraductal carcinomas of the breast (ductal carcinoma *in situ*) without true invasion are 'early' lesions, often multifocal and are increasingly discovered during mammographic screening. Breast cancer spreads lymphatically, both locally and to distant sites. Hematogenous spread occurs particularly to bone, liver, lung, skin and the central nervous system and can happen early during the course of the disease.

The diagnosis for a breast lump is established by clinical examination, mammography and/or ultrasound scan, and fine-needle aspiration biopsy or histology. Aspiration of cysts is easy and the finding of cysts with typical greenish fluid and disappearance of the lump after aspiration make the diagnosis of cancer extremely unlikely. Fine-needle aspiration cytology from solid lesions is established as a useful and accurate technique. If there is diagnostic uncertainty, a much larger piece of tissue can be obtained by core biopsy with a wide bore percutaneous biopsy needle, which usually yields an adequate core of tissue. Ultrasound-guided core needle biopsy, stereotactic biopsy and magnetic resonance imaging (MRI)-directed biopsy are important diagnostic tools, especially for women with suspicious but non-palpable breast masses. If a diagnosis cannot be reached after these investigations then excisional biopsy is necessary. Treatment options for breast cancer are surgery, radiotherapy, chemotherapy and hormonal manipulation.

Table 8.8 Risk stratification and survival rates for breast cancer

Group	Five-year survival (%)	Example	Treatment
Minimal risk (stage 1)	> 90	Screen-detected < 1 cm or ductal carcinoma *in situ*	Local
Low risk (stage 2)	70–90	Node negative, histologic grades I and II	Loco-regional
High risk (stage 2)	50–70	Node positive or histologic grade III	Loco-regional and systemic
Locally advanced (stage 3)	30–50	Large tumor or skin fixation/ulceration	Primary systemic
Metastatic (stage 4)	12–18	Skin, bone, lung, liver brain	Primary systemic

Prognosis depends on the stage, histologic grade and estrogen receptor (ER) status. Prognosis is best when there is no lymph node involvement and worse when four or more lymph nodes are affected. Treatment modalities and survival rates are outlined in Table 8.8. Breast cancer can recur many years after the initial diagnosis and treatment. Overall survival rates from all stages combined are 65% at 5, 35% at 10 and 30% at 15 years.

Hormone receptors in breast cancer

Normal breast cells have both estrogen and progesterone (PR) receptors. The breast estradiol receptor content is 5–10% of that in the endometrium. ERs are present in 65% of cancers in postmenopausal women, but only in 30% of cancers in premenopausal women. ER and PR positivity denotes that the tumor cells are better differentiated and have retained some of the features of the healthy cells. ER-positive breast cancers are more likely to respond to hormonal manipulation, thus oophorectomy can be avoided in patients who have ER-negative tumors. At most 5–7% of ER-negative tumors will respond to hormonal manipulation. Conversely, 30–40% of either ER- or PR-positive tumors will respond; when both receptors are present the rate is 70–90%. Tamoxifen reduces the risk of relapse and mortality by 25% and 17% at five years, respectively. Adjuvant tamoxifen taken for up to five years reduces the risks of recurrence and death in postmenopausal women independent of the ER status of the tumor, independently of nodal involvement or chemotherapy. The same is true for premenopausal women but only for those with ER-positive tumors. There is no additional benefit from extending treatment beyond five years and there is an increased risk of cancer of the endometrium and venous thromboembolism associated with tamoxifen treatment. For premenopausal women, ovarian ablation either by surgery or radiotherapy significantly improves survival, independent of lymph note status. If tamoxifen fails, aromatase inhibitors are used as second-line and progestins as third-line treatment. In hormone-resistant disease, chemotherapy is recommended.

Prevention of breast cancer

Tamoxifen and raloxifen substantially decrease the risk of breast cancer. This was shown in a recent major controlled trial with over 7000 participants demonstrating that in high risk women 20 mg/day tamoxifen for 4 years decreases the risk of breast cancer by a third. However, the routine prescription of these drugs for prevention has not yet become established clinical practice. Hemoprevention should be considered for individuals at high risk for breast cancer. Other preventative measures are: (1) decreasing alcohol and dietary fat intake; (2) increasing exercise; and (3) breastfeeding.

Screening for breast cancer

To screen or not to screen – that is the dilemma. The problem is not simply medical but also a matter of economics. To screen the entire adult female population on a regular basis is expensive. In healthcare systems, such as the NHS, it can only be justified if screening together with effective treatment of asymptomatic disease can be shown to reduce the mortality rates in a cost-effective manner.

Ideal criteria for establishing a screening program are set out in Table 8.9. Sadly, so far, there is no screening program which fulfills all these criteria.

The purpose of breast cancer screening is to distinguish women who are clearly normal from those with abnormality. The goal of breast cancer screening is to reduce morbidity and mortality caused by breast cancer. This is to be achieved by intervening in the disease process after biological onset but before symptoms develop. There are three methods for breast cancer screening that are currently practiced: X-ray mammography, clinical breast examination and breast self-examination.

Mammography

Breast cancer screening by mammography is the only screening procedure which has been evaluated by means of randomized controlled trials. Nevertheless, screening mammography has been more controversial than perhaps any other medical intervention. Provided that the intervention does not cause significant harm, we subscribe to the view that a treatment is effective until proven ineffective, in parallel with the well-established concept of innocent until proven guilty.

The most definitive measure of efficacy of a breast cancer screening program and the least subject to bias is the breast cancer *mortality rate* as determined by comparing screened and unscreened groups in randomized clinical

Table 8.9 Ideal criteria for establishing a screening program

Important health problem
Acceptable treatment available
Natural history understood
Recognizable latent phase
Suitable test available:
   simple
   acceptable
   accurate
   repeatable
   high sensitivity and specificity
Early treatment improves prognosis
Agreed policy on whom to treat
Effective diagnosis and treatment available
Case finding is a continuous, not one-off process
Cost of treating early disease substantially lower than
   cost of treating advanced disease

trials. *Survival*, in itself, does not establish that the natural history of the disease has been altered or that mortality has been reduced. Screening aims to detect breast cancer at a very early stage when cure is more likely. Mammography can detect cancers as small as 1 mm, which compares very favorably with clinical examination. Mammography does not have 100% accuracy and negative mammography does not mean that there is no cancer present. However, mammography detects over 90% of all breast cancers. Mammography and clinical examination are complementary and if there is strong suspicion of a palpable lesion, biopsy should be attempted even if the mammography is negative.

Single-view mammography uses a 1.2 mSv radiation exposure to the breast. The lifetime risk of induction of a cancer from one such examination in this age group is about 1:100 000. For women aged 40–49 this risk is approximately doubled. The risk of developing breast cancer naturally in any one year is about 120–150 per 100 000 women. The small carcinogenic risk of mammography is justified on the basis that mammographically detected cancers carry a greatly improved prognosis. Radiation exposures from widely

Table 8.10 Radiation exposure from various widely used diagnostic procedures

Diagnostic procedure	Typical radiation dose (mSv)	Approx. equiv. period of radiation from a natural background source
Chest (single postero-anterior film)	0.02	3 days
Hip	0.3	7 weeks
Abdomen	1.0	7 months
Mammography	1.2	8 months
Lung ventilation/perfusion scan	1.3	8 months
Computed tomography head scan	2.3	1 year
Barium enema	7	3.2 years

mSv, milli Sievent (unit of dose of ionizing radiation which delivers one joule of energy per kg recipient mass)

used diagnostic procedures are outlined in Table 8.10.

Screening in the UK is performed by inviting all women aged between 50 and 64 years to undergo a mammography every three years. The first screen consists of a two-view mammography, and subsequent mammograms are performed by a single-view (in a two-view mammography the projections are cranioaural and mediolateral, whereas in a single-view mammography there is only an oblique mediolateral view). Practices vary between countries. For example, in the USA, mammography is recommended every year after the age of 40 years, while in Sweden every 18–24 months is the standard recommendation. In both countries two-view mammography is the norm. The optimum age group to be screened and frequency of mammography remain uncertain but it is thought that screening decreases mortality by 20–25%[1,2,3].

When a screening program begins, about 10–20 prevalent cases are detected per 1000 women. At follow-up, the new incident case rate is about 2–6 per 1000 women per year. Of all mammographically detected cancers, 20% are *in situ* disease and 40% are less than 1 cm in diameter. Overall around 65% are less than 2 cm in diameter. This compares very favorably with clinically detected cancers, where barely one-quarter are 2 cm or less. Cancers less then 2 cm in diameter which have no lymph node involvement carry the best prognosis. When there is an invasive lesion as opposed to *in situ*, there is always a possibility of metastasis. Once the tumor is over 5 cm in diameter, a cure is unlikely. Currently, 90% of women who are referred for further investigation upon screening do not have cancer, and this point should be stressed to minimize anxiety. The effectiveness of mammographic screening depends, amongst other things, on the total number of women attending regularly for screening. Currently the uptake for screening is between 55 and 90%, depending on education, social class, age and area of the country. A downside of breast cancer screening is that it generates additional work for staff and anxiety in some women. In addition, some of the *in situ* cancers may not become clinically significant in the lifetime of the woman.

Breast self-examination

More than 80% of clinically diagnosed breast cancers are discovered as a lump by the patient. Intuitively it follows that regular breast self-examination may help discover some cancers at an earlier stage, when the prognosis is more favorable. However, less research has been devoted to clinical breast examination and/or breast self-examination than to mammography. Breast self-examination should probably start after the age of 35 years. Women should be taught by a well-trained practitioner. The stages of examination are as follows:

(1) The woman should undress to the waist and stand in front of a mirror, carefully looking at all parts of both breasts, first with her arms relaxed, then stretched over her head. Then she should put her hands on her hips and watch the breasts when she presses her hands into her hips and relaxes.

(2) The woman should be looking for any difference in shape between the breasts. Size is not important because often one breast is bigger than the other. She should be looking for changes with arm movements and when her hands are pressed against her hips. With early cancer, there can be slight depression, flattening, rippling or dimpling of the skin in one part of one breast. The nipple may become deviated or become depressed or retracted. These changes can occur in very early cancers when there is no lump to feel. Tethering or peau d'orange are signs associated with both early and advanced disease and can be seen in any position.

(3) Palpation of all areas of both breasts, including the axillary tail, should be covered and any new differences between the two sides should be reported. Cancers under 2 cm are not usually the 'cherry stones' that most women expect. They could be just a bit of thickening with a slight depression when the pectoral muscles are contracted. However, tumors usually feel harder than they are, due to involvement of the surrounding tissue.

(4) Any new symptoms should be reported. A blood-stained nipple discharge is very worrying to the woman, but the majority are benign and are due to either duct papillomas or duct ectasias. One-sided and particularly serous discharges from one duct of one nipple should be reported to the doctor, as should the development of localized discomfort or an odd, strange feeling which is often localized and difficult to describe but which does not resemble premenstrual tenderness.

(5) Monthly self-examination, after menstruation, is ideal.

There are now several epidemiologic studies indicating that survival is increased in women practicing breast self-examination and that cancers detected by breast self-examination tend to be smaller. However, as discussed earlier, an increase in survival does not necessarily translate into reduction in the mortality rates. Although these results are promising, firm evidence that the mortality rate is reduced is lacking and more data are needed.

Clinical breast examination

Clinical breast examination (CBE) has not been adequately tested against an unexamined control group, and there is no experimental evidence that the benefit of annual breast examination exceeds the possible harm resulting from false-negative and false-positive examination. Not surprisingly, recommendations regarding CBE vary. In the UK, the Department of Health (the government's advisory committee on breast cancer screening) has advised that breast palpation should not be included as part of routine health screening. However, the Canadian Task Force on periodic health examination, the US Preventive Services Task Force and the American College of Physicians all recommend yearly CBE starting from the age of 40 years. It is a well known fact that the mortality from breast cancer in the US is lower than that in the UK. To what extent, if any, CBE is contributing to the lower mortality is still matter of debate.

When performed by carefully trained medical personnel, CBE is quoted to have a sensitivity of 80% and specificity of 88–96% at the first examination[4]. These figures may look overoptimistic and non-attainable in everyday clinical practice; however, on the other hand, they clearly show the potential of CBE.

ACKNOWLEDGEMENTS

This chapter was extensively reviewed by Dr J. Steel, Consultant, Breast Screening Service, and Dr L. Chapman, Department of Surgery, both at Derifford Hospital, Plymouth, UK.

References

1. Nyström L, Andersson I, Bjurstam N, *et al*. Long-term effects of mammography screening: updated overview of the Swedish randomised trials. *Lancet* 2002;359:909–19
2. Tabar L, Yen MF, Vitak B, *et al*. Mammography service screening and mortality in breast cancer patients; 20-year follow-up before and after introduction of screening. *Lancet 2003* 361: 1405–10
3. Otto SJ, Fracheboud J, Looman CW, *et al*. Initiation of population-based mammography screening in Dutch municipalities and effect on breast cancer mortality: a systematic review. *Lancet* 2003;361:1411–7
4. Rimer BK. Breast cancer screening. In Harris JR, *et al.*, ed. *Diseases of the Breast*. Philadelphia, PA: Lippincott 1996:318

Sexual function and dysfunction 9

Nikolai Manassiev

INTRODUCTION

Sexuality is an important component of physical, intellectual, psychologic and social well-being. This central role of sexuality in a person's life is affected by health or illness and by many psychologic factors. Physicians have the opportunity to assess the sexual function in the course of routine history taking; however, this is rarely done. Additionally, many doctors are uncomfortable with the patient's questions about sexuality and feel uneasy about broaching the subject themselves. In some cases, they feel that such questions are an intrusion on the patient's privacy, even though they realize that bowel and drug habits, cigarette and alcohol use and reproductive status are also private matters. In other cases, they believe that the patient's sexual concerns are not of medical significance or that their own ability to treat such concerns is limited. In this way, they ignore or dismiss the patient's concerns.

Patients may expect their physician to be an authority on sexual matters but frequently are unable to express their concerns for fear of being criticized or misunderstood. Surveys of clinical practices show that only 10% of patients will initiate a discussion of sexual problems if the physician does not, but over 50% will describe a sexual concern if the doctor provides an opportunity for discussion. Thus, the onus of breaking the vicious circle of avoiding talking about sexual matters seems to fall on the physician. Such enquiry may lead to a diagnostic clue in an otherwise elusive diagnosis.

Concerns about sexual matters and sexual dysfunctions affect all ages. It is important to remember that the demographics of the Western societies are changing. There is an increase in longevity, which leads to two separate phenomena. On the one hand, there is a large population of middle and retirement age people who are spared the ravages of harsh physical labor, and who age in good general health with a secure income. On the other hand, many patients with previously untreatable chronic diseases, such as cancer, hypertension, angina, diabetes, depression, rheumatoid arthritis and osteoarthritis, live much longer with an improved prognosis. In both groups, the presence of a sexual dysfunction may completely spoil the enjoyment of better health. Therefore, it is necessary that health professionals nowadays should have a basic understanding of human sexuality and sexual dysfunctions.

HUMAN SEXUAL RESPONSE

Procreation through sexual activity is an adaptive evolutional response, which gives the species a high potential for survival. Sexual behavior – a much wider subject – is, however, a learned behavior. In mammals and non-human primates, it is controlled by instincts with timing dependent on the estrus cycle of the female. By contrast human sexual behavior is influenced by the family, sociologic factors (mass media, community institutions and social milieu), individual experience and choice.

Even though sexual behavior and attitudes toward sex vary greatly among individuals, the desire for sexual pleasure is thought to be strong in most men and women. It should be noted that sex for satisfying sexual hunger is only one reason for sexual experience. Other reasons for having sex with a partner, and particularly important for women, are: (1) to enhance emotional closeness, bonding, commitment, sharing and tolerance; (2) to show love and affection; or (3) to let the partner see that he/she has been missed (emotionally and/or physically). There is no consensus regarding terminology for the force that makes us initiate or respond to sexual behavior, but commonly used terms for it are *libido*, *sex drive* and *sexual desire*. Another definition of libido is: the force by which sexual instinct is represented in the mind. Libido is a word of Latin origin and means pleasure, lust, desire.

Some researchers make a distinction between sex drive and sexual desire. For them sex drive is an omnipotent force that can lead to all forms of sexual outlet: sexual fantasies, masturbation, intercourse. Sexual desire is defined as the sexual drive toward a particular sexual outlet, i.e., intercourse with husband in preference to masturbation. This divide may be quite unnecessary and most people (professionals or lay) use libido, sex drive and sexual desire interchangeably. The frequency and intensity of sexual desire and sexual activity and the degree of sexual satisfaction vary throughout one's life. Nevertheless, the phases of the sexual response cycle remain the same and do not change. Meaningful discussion about sexual dysfunction is impossible without being thoroughly familiar with the phases of the sexual response.

Phases of the sexual response cycle

The phases of human sexual response are sexual desire, arousal (excitement), orgasm and resolution (Table 9.1).

Desire

This phase is characterized by sexual fantasies and the desire to have sexual activity. It is distinct from other phases because it is psychological and reflects motivations, drives and personality.

Arousal (excitement)

The physiologic purpose of sexual arousal is two-fold: (1) to facilitate the painless penetration of the vagina by the penis and to reduce the risk of discomfort and trauma during sexual intercourse; and (2) to induce a pleasure response which will motivate an individual to seek sexual activity on another occasion. Sexual arousal is dependent on sexual stimuli, of which there are two types: those dependent on the brain (psychic), such as sight (visual), sound (auditory), smell (olfactory) and sexual fantasies, and those dependent on touch (reflexive). The latter can be effective independent of the brain, e.g., following spinal cord transection. The most powerful of these stimuli is touch, especially of the erogenous areas of the body. There is a wide variability between persons and within the same person in sensitivity to sexual stimuli, which may be under biochemical, hormonal, circadian or social influence.

Sexual stimulation leads to central and peripheral arousal and genital response. Central arousal is the state of alertness that focuses the attention on sexual stimulation. Peripheral arousal is increased sensitivity to touch. In the female, genital responses include local vasocongestion, vaginal lubrication, clitoral erection, uterine elevation and increased muscle tone. Local vasocongestion leads to eversion of labia majora and minora, thereby facilitating penile penetration. As a result of increased tone of the pubococcygeal muscle, the lower third of the vagina 'narrows' and the upper third widens and elongates. The uterus occupies a higher position in the pelvis and the moisture of the secretions facilitates penile entry and thrusting. The neural pathways controlling these changes are via the parasympathetic sacral outflow of S2–S4 via the nervi erigentes. In addition, there is involvement in the sympathetic nervous system leading to increased alertness, rise of pulse and blood pressure.

Orgasm and resolution

It is difficult to define orgasm but two such attempts described it as an 'explosive discharge of neuromuscular tension' or simply as 'piercing sexual pleasure'. In the female, a few seconds after the start of orgasm, there is a

Table 9.1 Female sexual response cycle

Parameter	Excitement phase	Orgasmic phase	Resolution phase
Time interval	Several minutes to several hours	3–25 s	10–15 min if orgasm; if no orgasm 0.5 h to 1 day
Skin	Inconsistent sexual flush: maculopapular rash may appear on abdomen, anterior chest, neck, face	Well-developed flush	Flush disappears. Inconsistent perspiration on palms and soles
Breasts	Nipple erection in two-thirds of women; areola enlargement. Breast size increases by 25%	Breasts may become tremulous	Return to normal size within an hour
Clitoris	Enlargement in diameter of glans and shaft	No changes	Detumescence in 5–30 min; if no orgasm, several hours
Labia majora	Congestion and edema. Eversion	No change	Return to normal size in 1–15 min
Labia minora	Congestion, size increases 2–3 times. Eversion. Color change to deep red	Contraction of proximal labia minora	Return to normal within 5 min
Bartholin's glands	Secretion		
Vagina	Color: dark purple. Lubrication, ballooning of upper third, constriction of lower third prior to orgasm.	3–15 contractions of the lower third	Congestion disappears in seconds. If no orgasm, in 20–30 min
Uterus	Elevation in the pelvis	Contractions throughout orgasm	Return to normal position
Rectum		Rhythmic contractions of anal sphincter	
Others	Myotonia	Loss of voluntary muscle control	Return to baseline

spasm of the muscles surrounding the lower third of the vagina, known as the orgasmic platform, followed by between five and eight rhythmic contractions. In some women, anal and uterine contractions are also observed. Orgasm is a sympathetic reflex, and during orgasm there is a rise in pulse rate (up to 160 beats per minute), blood pressure (both systolic and diastolic: by 20–40 mmHg), respiration rate and pupillary dilation. Orgasm lasts between 3 and 25 s and may be associated with a slight clouding of consciousness. After the orgasm, a period of calm follows which is termed resolution. Various surveys suggest that 30–50% of women experience orgasm from coitus, a larger number from clitoral stimulation, and 10–20% do not experience orgasm in spite of being highly aroused sexually. It appears that orgasm in women is not a purely reflexive event as in men but is more of a learned ability. The number of women able to experience orgasm increases with age. In adolescence only 50% of women experience orgasm; this increases to 95% by age 35. In women, the refractory period is not very well defined and some even question

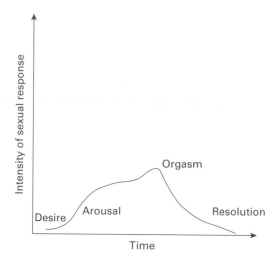

Figure 9.1 Diagram of the sexual response cycle

its existence. Kinsey reports that 14% of women are capable of experiencing multiple orgasms. The time course of sexual responses in the female is longer than in the male. A summary of the body changes during the sexual response cycle is provided in Table 9.1. Figure 9.1 represents the phases of the sexual response cycle.

The sexual response is a unique blend of psychologic and physiologic experiences. Psychosexual development, attitudes toward sexuality and the sexual partner are directly involved with, and affect, the nature of human sexual response (Table 9.2).

Stress is a pervasive cause of sexual problems. Difficulties at work, unemployment, money concerns, worries over children and interpersonal conflicts all contribute to sexual problems. The presence of relationship problems is one of the most damaging types of stress as the source of the stress and the sexual partner are the same person. An example of relationship problems is excessive politeness and consideration, presenting with a low level of sexual activity, vaginismus or impotence. Another example is when the couple has different sexual attitudes or different sexual desires. In some couples, there is a protective realtionship problem. It happens when one of

the partners who does not enjoy sex at the best of times is protecting the sicker partner from the stresses of sex on spurious medical grounds. We should not forget extramarital affairs, which may lead to a lack of desire in the partner who feels betrayed.

Most psychiatric conditions can lead to sexual problems. It is amply documented that depression leads to decreased motivation and sex drive. In anxiety states sexual problems are common. In schizophrenia the libido may be preserved, but interpersonal relationship problems inhibit sexual activity.

Poor general health, notably peripheral vascular disease and diabetes, through decreased vascular response and sensitivity, may lead to an insufficient sexual response. For some, the rigor of sex may be too much a demand for the rest of the body, even if there is a desire and genital response.

Excess alcohol may cause (1) low levels of testosterone; (2) neuropathy and decreased genital sensitivity; (3) hypertension; (4) depression; and (5) jealousy and partnership problems. In addition, the intoxicated partner may be clumsy, smelly or demanding. In drug addiction, the sphere of interest can be so narrow as to exclude everything else but drugs. Aversion to sex is well documented in people who have experienced sexual abuse in childhood or rape.

An excessively rigid and cold upbringing can be particularly destructive for a person's sex life. On the one hand, it may lead to promiscuity, where the person seeks substitutes for love and affection and reassurance; on the other hand, it may lead to decreased desire and arousal and the view that sex is dirty.

Aging and the sexual response

The speed and intensity of the vasocongestive response decreases with aging. There is a reduction in the elasticity of the vaginal wall and the size of the vagina itself. Vaginal lubrication is slower and less marked and breast changes are less noticeable. Orgasm in older women is associated with fewer contractions and occasionally may be painful. The

Table 9.2 Some factors affecting sexual response

Stress
Age
Relationship with partner
Physical and mental health
Sexual knowledge/education
Self-image and confidence
Sexual experiences
Sexual attitudes/values
Parental influence/attitude
Sexual novelty/boredom
Drug/alcohol addiction

Table 9.3 Factors associated with aging that adversely affect sexual response

Physical deconditioning
Chronic disease(s)
Increased use of medication
Age-related emotional problems
Situational
   widowhood
   nursing home environment
Expectations
   society
   personal
Previously low sexual activity

resolution phase is more rapid in older women. These changes become increasingly prominent after the menopause and some are related to estrogen and/or testosterone deficiency. There is an increased latency to excitement and greater need for longer tactile stimulation and an increased refractory period (Table 9.3). Longitudinal data show that, for healthy women, aging is not associated with decreased sexual desire or decreased orgasmic capacity. Aging may be associated with quantitative but not qualitative changes in sexual activity.

Epidemiologic observations

Large-scale observations of human sexuality were started by Alfred Kinsey and co-workers in the United States in 1941. Their work was expanded in 1947 with the founding of the Kinsey Institute. Kinsey was professor of zoology at Indiana University, when, in 1938, he was asked to teach marriage preparation classes. It was then that he realized how little truly scientific data existed on human sexual behavior. More than 18 000 interviews were conducted and a tremendous amount of data collected. Many original observations and publications on human sexual response, function and dysfunction as well as sexual behavior were based on these data. Many of these observations are still true today, but some are not because (1) the methodology used was not

appropriate; (2) sexual behavior is a biological, psychologic and social phenomenon – as the society changes so do some aspects of sexuality.

Kinsey noted that in men social class is an important determinant of sexual behavior. Working-class men would experience sexual intercourse at an early age and engage much less in petting and oral sex. Once married, they would become involved in extramarital affairs early on in the marriage, but less so when getting older. Upper-class men would be more likely to engage in petting and oral sex. They tended to be faithful until middle age, when they might seek extramarital opportunities.

For women, social class was found to have a smaller impact on sexual behavior. Kinsey noted that some women could go through long periods of sexual inactivity. He concluded that men are more responsive to psychologic stimuli (fantasies and visual cues), while women require more tactile stimulation, though they also respond to visual, sexually explicit material. Kinsey reported that almost all men and 75% of women had masturbated at some stage in their lives.

Research into the epidemiology of sexual function continues, and the results of two cross-sectional studies of women in the UK and the United States are presented in Table 9.4. The UK study found that sexual interest in women varies across social classes. Impaired sexual interest was reported by 12%

Table 9.4 Results of two cross-sectional studies investigating sexual disorders in women in the UK and the United States

Problem	Study 1 (%)*	Study 2 (%)**
Impaired sexual interest	17	30
Impaired arousal	17	21
Impaired orgasm	16	25
Dyspareunia	8	16
Any sexual dysfunction	33	43
Sex not pleasurable	–	19
Anxiety about performance	–	11
Help seeking	4	20

*Comprising 436 sexually active women aged between 35 and 59 years; **comprising 1749 sexually active women aged between 18 and 59 years

of classes I–II; 18% in class III; and 15% in classes IV–V. There was no correlation of sexual dysfunction to menopausal symptoms. A history of psychiatric problems was reported by 10% of those reporting sexual dysfunction. Age, marital problems and neurotic predisposition were identified in 72% of cases. Interestingly, even though 33% of participants were found to have some form of sexual dysfunction, only 10% identified themselves as having sexual problems, and this was not related to age. Even more remarkable, only 4% said that they would commence treatment if available. The American study found that single people were more likely to have an orgasmic disorder than married ones. High educational attainment was found to be associated with fewer sexual problems in both sexes. Risk factors for sexual problems were stress and a deteriorating economic position (expressed as a decline in household income). Arousal disorders were frequently found in women with adult–child sexual contact or forced sexual contact. Sexual problems were more prevalent in younger women and older men.

One American cross-sectional study of adults aged 60–85 years found that 69% of men and 30% of women were sexually active, married ones more so than unmarried ones. Among married couples 74% of men and 56% of women were sexually active. The corresponding figure for single individuals was 31% for men and 5% for women. Sexual activity correlated with incontinence, poor mobility, heart problems and sedatives. Among married men, 30–65% were impotent, depending on age.

It is evident from many studies that the main sexual problem in women is lack of desire, while in men it is erectile dysfunction.

SEXUAL HISTORY

In medicine, history and examination are the cornerstones on which diagnoses and treatment strategies are made. In the field of sexual medicine, history is of paramount importance.

Proper history taking requires a lot of time. Time is limited in outpatient clinics and surgeries and that is why history taking has to be shortened and concentrated on clarifying the presenting complaints and on the relevant background features. The doctor should not be embarrassed, otherwise the patient may retract or deviate from the topic. Openness, good communication skills and tact encourage and promote frank discussion.

The presenting complaint should be explored in detail regarding its nature, development and duration and the role of situational factors. Bearing in mind the nature of the sexual response in women, questions should be asked regarding the presence of sexual desire or aversion to sex, adequacy of lubrication, the partner's ability to penetrate, reaction to penetration, pain during or after sexual intercourse and the ability to achieve orgasm. Questions should be asked about the partner's sexual desire, quality of erection, orgasm and ejaculation. Those about sexual knowledge and expectations are very relevant: for example, the patient may not be aware that coital frequency varies considerably and tends to decrease with age and with the length of a relationship. Questions regarding the quality and duration of the current relationship, previous relationships, separation and infidelities should come next. Then comes sexual development, sexual experiences

Table 9.5 Areas that should be covered by the sexual history

Nature and development of the sexual problem
Sexual knowledge and expectations
Relationship with partner
  development
  sexual relationship
  general relationship
  children and contraception
  infidelity
  commitment
Sexual experience (positive/negative/traumatic)
Medical history (e.g., diabetes, heart disease)
Surgical history (e.g., pelvic or genital operations)
Psychiatric history (e.g., depression)
Alcohol, drug and tobacco use
Appearance and mood
Attitude to problem and treatment

Table 9.6 Common sexual dysfunctions

Sexual desire disorders
  hypoactive sexual desire
  sexual aversion/avoidance
Sexual arousal disorders
Orgasmic disorders
Sexual pain disorders
  dyspareunia
  vaginismus

(positive/negative/traumatic) and masturbation. The important points in taking a sexual history are summarized in Table 9.5.

Inquiries about general medical, psychiatric and drug history will help in assessing the possibility of an organic, psychologic or drug-induced condition(s). It is essential to keep in mind the possibility of depression and to ask specific questions about mood, appetite, sleeping pattern, etc. The doctor should attempt to form some impression about the character and personality of the patient. At the end of the consultation the doctor should ask about the degree by which the problem causes personal distress or strain to the relationship. Genital examination and general physical examination should be performed only if clinically indicated and with caution if there is a history of sexual abuse. A chaperone should always be present and the option of a male or female doctor should be offered if possible. Women with vaginismus may be very reluctant to be examined and only agree to this over time, once trust has been established and they can remain in control.

COMMON SEXUAL PROBLEMS

The classification of sexual dysfunction follows the pattern of sexual response and a simplified version is given in Table 9.6. It is of paramount importance to note that for a disorder to be diagnosed the mere presence of a condition is not enough; it must also cause personal distress. For example, we cannot diagnose hypoactive sexual desire in a woman who reports no sexual fantasies but is not troubled by it. Each of the diagnoses in Table 9.6 is subclassified as (1) life-long versus acquired; (2) generalized versus situational; and (3) etiologic/organic, psychogenic, mixed or unknown.

Problems of sexual response

Any part of the female sexual response can be affected. It is useful to have some working definitions when attempting to evaluate and help women.

Sexual desire disorders

Low sexual desire If a woman can generate sexual fantasies and daydreams or if she masturbates, then by definition her sexual desire is intact. If, however, there is a lack of thoughts about sex or masturbation, or a lack of responsiveness to her partner's initiation, then sexual desire is said to be impaired. An estimated 17–30% (depending on the population studied) of women have a hypoactive sexual desire disorder. Often, women presenting with low sexual desire disclose that their partner's desire is higher than their own. The presenting problem then is discrepant sexual desire. However, sexual activity may still be present even if sexual desire is low. For example, many women are sexually active – but only to please their partner or to preserve the relationship. It has been reported that for 6% of women sex is an obligation rather than an enjoyable activity. Such women are defined as having a low pro-activity (not seeking sexual behavior) but an intact receptivity (ability to respond to sexual advances). The presence of desire depends on several factors: biological drive, good sexual experiences, the availability of a partner and a good relationship in non-sexual areas. Damage to any of these factors may result in decreased desire. Other factors that can suppress sexual desire are depressants of the central nervous system, abstinence from sex for a prolonged period of time, major illness or an affected body image (mastectomy, ileostomy, colostomy, hysterectomy or vulvectomy).

Inhibition of desire may be a defensive way of protecting against unconscious fear of sex or pregnancy. Loss of desire may also be an expression of hostility or the sign of a deteriorating relationship. It is important to establish a baseline of sexual interest before the disorder began because sexual activity varies among people (one study found that 8% of couples have intercourse less than once a month). The diagnosis should not be made unless the lack of desire is a source of distress to the patient.

Sexual aversion disorders Sexual aversion disorders are defined as a persistent or recurrent extreme aversion to, and avoidance of, all or almost all genital sexual contact with a sexual partner. This condition goes beyond the simple avoidance of sexual activity to include sexual panic states, sexual aversion and sexual phobias. Some of these patients may have a normal sex drive and sexual fantasies, and be able to enjoy autoerotic activity, but when confronted with a sexual partner in a sexual situation, they may experience aversion to the partner's touch or to contact with the partner's genitalia or semen.

Impaired sexual excitement (arousal)

Problems with sexual excitement present as either an inadequate physiologic response to sexual stimulation (lubrication, swelling, etc.) or a lack of sense of pleasurable feeling during sexual stimulation. It is thought to present in about 20% of patients. Women who have impaired sexual arousal often have orgasm problems as well. Sexual arousal naturally fluctuates, with some women reporting greatest sexual excitement immediately after a period and others at the time of ovulation. Impairment with physiologic excitement can be recognized by the lack of genital changes in response to effective sexual stimulation. It should be noted that some women do not register that genital changes have occured when in fact they have. Changes in testosterone, estrogen, prolactin and thyroxin levels have been implicated in arousal disorders. The progestogenic effect of the progestogen-only pill, antihistamine and anti-cholinergic medications can cause a decrease in vaginal lubrication. An insufficient genital response may simply be due to inadequate sexual stimulation. The lack of pleasurable feeling during sexual stimulation is more likely to be psychologic, and numerous psychologic factors are associated with sexual inhibition (Table 9.7). These conflicts may be expressed through inhibition of excitement or orgasm and are discussed in the section on Orgasmic disorders, below. However, decrease in sensitivity in erogenous areas may occur with hormonal deficiencies (Table 9.8).

Orgasmic disorders (anorgasmia)

Anorgasmia is an inability to achieve orgasm by masturbation or coitus and this accounts for approximately 5% of sexual disorders. A futher 15–20% report dissatisfaction with the quality of their orgasms. It can be an isolated problem with sexual desire and arousal being intact. Often, however, excitement and orgasmic disorders coexist and share the same etiology. Anorgasmia may be situational, i.e., more commonly present with the partner and not with masturbation (i.e., many women are orgasmic with manual stimulation but not during coitus). Orgasm during coitus may be achieved by the combination of manual clitoral stimulation and penile vaginal stimulation.

Table 9.7 Summary of psychologic causes of sexual dysfunction

Deteriorating relationship – anger/boredom/habituation
Depression
Lack of
  trust between partners
  communication with the partner about sex
  sex for a prolonged period of time
  knowledge about sex organs and their function
Aging
Fears of
  pregnancy
  intimacy/dependency/rejection
  partner's genitals/semen
  loss of control
  performance failure
  painful sex
Physiologic changes: transition to motherhood
Loss of fertility (i.e., early menopause)
Inhibitory factors
  guilt after pleasurable experience/masturbation
  religious upbringing/cultural expectations/societal restriction
  trauma: forceful sex/rape/incest
  belief in sexual myths, e.g., nice girls don't initiate sex
Bereavement/grief

Table 9.8 Summary of organic and iatrogenic causes of female sexual response disorders

a) Organic causes

Endocrine
Estrogen deficiency
Testosterone deficiency
Diabetes
Hyperprolactinemia
Hypothyroidism
Hypopituitarism
Addison's disease
Cushing's disease

Neurologic
Spinal cord conditions (i.e., multiple sclerosis, trauma)
Epilepsy
Stroke
Lumbar canal stenosis
Head injury
Tumor

Substance abuse
Alcohol
Drugs

b) Iatrogenic

Surgical
Mastectomy and other disfiguring surgery,
  e.g., colostomy
Sympathectomy
Retroperitoneal lymphadenopathy/lymphadenectomy
Pelvic/vaginal surgery

Induced premature menopause
Surgery
Radiotherapy
Chemotherapy

Medications
Dopamine antagonists
Sedatives
Hypnotics
Antidepressants (fluoxetine, monoamine oxidase
  inhibitors, tricyclic antidepressants)
Anxiolytics
α-Adrenoreceptor antagonists
Combined oral contraceptives
Antiandrogens

Primary orgasmic dysfunction exists when the woman has never experienced orgasm with any sort of stimulation. Secondary orgasmic dysfunction exists if the woman has experienced at least one orgasm regardless of circumstances or means of stimulation. According to Kinsey, the first orgasm occurs during adolescence in about 50% of women, and this proportion increases as women get older. Kinsey found that the proportion of married women over 35 years old who had never achieved orgasm by any means was only 5%. Increased orgasmic potential in women over 35 has been explained on the basis of less psychologic inhibition or greater sexual experience, or both. Orgasmic dysfunction is a common complaint. A number of psychologic, organic and iatrogenic factors are associated with inhibited female orgasms (Tables 9.7 and 9.8).

Sexual pain disorders

Vaginismus is an involuntary contraction of the pelvic floor muscles and outer third of the vagina, making penetration impossible or very painful. It is usually a psychologic problem, being a phobia of vaginal penetration. For example, a phobic response may be triggered by painful sex (especially forceful

Table 9.9 Common causes of painful intercourse

Superficial pain
Vulvovaginal atrophy
Episiotomy
Tight skin bridge or fissure at the fourchette
Infections
   herpes
   genital warts
   candidiasis
   trichomoniasis
   bartholinitis
Dermatologic conditions
   allergy/irritations
   eczema
   lichen sclerosus
   psoriasis
Vulvovaginal surgery
Cystocele
Vestibulitis
Lack of lubrication

Deep pain
Constipation
Endometriosis
Postoperative adhesions
Pelvic inflammatory disease
Fibroids
Inflammatory bowel disease
Ovarian cysts
Cystitis

Superficial and deep pain estrogen deficiency

sex), fear of pregnancy, or a strict religious upbringing.

Dyspareunia means genital pain during or after intercourse. The pain may be superficial, involving the vulva, the introitus and the lower third of the vagina, or deep, when it is felt near the cervix or the lower abdominal area. Vaginismus and dyspareunia are closely linked as vaginismus may be a cause of superficial pain and dyspareunia may result in protective vaginismus reflex. Common pathologic causes of painful intercourse are listed in Table 9.9.

Vulvar vestibulitis is inflammation of the vestibular glands, which are mucous-secreting glands. These glands are arranged concentrically around the introitus between the labia minora and the hymen. Should they become inflamed, they lead to dyspareunia with penetration, pruritus and erythema. On inspection there may be erythema at the area and the vestibular glands may be raised, giving a rough (uneven) appearance. Probing with a cottonwool swab reveals an exquisite tenderness (point tenderness).

DIAGNOSIS AND MANAGEMENT

Although approaches to treatment of sexual dysfunction vary, some general principles are applicable. The careful taking of a history, an appropriate clinical examination and investigations should help distinguish between organic and psychogenic causes (Tables 9.7 and 9.8). Although there are no controlled research studies of most sexual dysfunctions, it is estimated that 60–80% are of psychogenic origin, marital disharmony and depression being the commonest. Once such a differentiation is made, appropriate treatment can be instituted. We see the role of the non-specialist as threefold. First, ruling out organic disease and assessing a contributing physical illness (arthritis, radical mastectomy, stroke, heart attack, etc.). Second, identifying psychologic factors, either as a primary cause for dysfunction or contributing to an organic cause. Third, eliciting discussion and educating the patient. The clinician should assist the patient in understanding the basis of the human sexual response and the intricate interplay between the physiologic and psychologic components. Open discussion about sexual matters can dispel many fears, anxieties or misinformation. Many patients have never had an opportunity to discuss their sexual experiences with a health professional. Breaking the barrier of silence, reducing anger and improving communication between partners may be sufficient for some patients. The doctor needs to assess the motivation of the patient/couple because treatment often requires considerable investment of time and effort.

A detailed description of the treatments is beyond the scope of this book and only selected treatments are going to be discussed. We believe that the patient should be given practical advice and treatment where possible but if (1) the diagnosis is in doubt; (2) the problem is too difficult; (3) there is poor rapport; or (4) there is no response, prompt referral to a psychosexual clinic should be made. Organic causes for sexual response disorders, painful penetration and painful sex should be treated accordingly. Depression needs to be excluded. If the problem persists in spite of accurate diagnosis and adequate treatment, it may be that the pathology cannot be fully resolved or there are coexisting psychologic factors. Strategies to cope with the problem, rather than a complete cure, may be more realistic.

Disorders of desire are the most difficult to treat. As mentioned above, educating the patient about a decline in desire with age, habituation, stress and relationship difficulties is important. A common sense suggestion, also applicable for arousal disorders, is setting time aside for relaxation; the need for warmth and perhaps flowers, scents, music, lubricants and in some cases sex aides.

Possible therapeutic avenues are pharmacologic doses of testosterone, HRT in postmenopausal women, apomorphine, buproprion, yohimbine. Of those only the first two have been shown to be effective.

Because a sexual arousal disorder almost invariably leads to an orgasmic disorder, the treatment of both disorders is similar. Counseling is very important. It should explore the relationship and its strengths, the domestic situation, occupation (e.g., shift work) and stressful life situations, etc. (Table 9.7).

Possible pharmacologic treatments are sildenafil, apomorphine, topical prostaglandins, testosterone and hormone replacement therapy (HRT) in postmenopausal women. The first three are promising, but unproven; the latter two are the effective ones.

The Masters and Johnson sensate focus exercises, in which the couple moves stepwise from non-genital pleasuring to genital pleasuring to non-demanding coitus, generally benefit women regardless of the level of sexual inhibition. Education should be provided regarding the function of the genital organs, sexual responses and the best methods of stimulating the clitoris and the vagina. Kegel's exercises strengthen voluntary control of the pelvic floor muscle. The muscles are contracted 10–15 times three times a day. Alternatively women are advised to do their pelvic floor exercises each time they pass urine – so it becomes simple routine. In two to three months, perivaginal muscle tone improves, as do the woman's sense of control and the quality of the orgasm.

The standard treatment of vaginismus consists of self-exploration by looking at and feeling the genitals, information about genital anatomy and the physiology of arousal, learning relaxation techniques, pelvic floor exercises, discussing the problem with the partner, stopping attempts at penetrative sex, and gradual vaginal dilation until confidence is rebuilt. Dyspareunia may also be relieved by the use of artificial lubricants, or by the changing of sexual position to one where penetration is limited (side by side) or controlled (the woman on top).

PREGNANCY AND THE PUERPERIUM

There are two special situations which warrant further discussion: pregnancy and puerperium and the menopause. Sexual activity during pregnancy decreases from 85% in the first trimester to 23% in the 36th week. Common reasons are physical discomfort, loss of interest and fear of injuring the fetus. After delivery, sexual activity resumes in three months for most couples. However, 50% of mothers and 15% of fathers report lower sexual desire and 60% of couples have less sexual activity at one year after delivery of the baby. The main reasons for this decline in sexual activity are summarized in Table 9.10.

All these factors need to be addressed in a simple and practical manner before extensive investigations are undertaken and before the couple is labeled as suffering from sexual dysfunction.

MENOPAUSE

Specific features of sexuality in the perimenopause and the menopause are given in Table 9.11.

Table 9.10 Causes for decline in sexual activity in the puerperium

Breastfeeding causing
  raised prolactin and low estrogen
  milk release on arousal
  time-consuming
Pain
  episiotomy
  tear
  Cesarean scar
Change of role to mother
Weight gain and poor body image
Fear of pregnancy
Exhaustion
Disturbed sleep pattern

Table 9.11 Factors contributing to sexual dysfunction in the menopause

Aging and its effects: dry skin, brittle hair, dry mucosae, painful joints, muscles
Pendulous breasts with increased fat content
Redistribution of body fat, especially to the buttock and abdomen (middle-aged spread)
Vasomotor symptoms
Sex hormone deficiency affecting
  sexual desire
  arousal
  lubrication
  congestion
  orgasm
Reaction to changed body image
Attitude to menopause
Marital relationship
Support network and coping with midlife crises
Society emphasis on youth and slimness

Table 9.12 Counseling women regarding testosterone implantation

50 mg implant over 6 months equals approximately 0.27 mg/day, which is similar to the natural production rate of testosterone
Adverse side-effects include
  oily skin
  acne
  altered lipid profile
  hirsutism
  alopecia
  voice changes

The psychologic and sociocultural dimensions need to be addressed in their own right. Adequate explanation about the process of aging and its effects on sexual dysfunction goes a long way. Most middle-aged and older people would not expect themselves to be as fit or to look as well as when they were young; however, some retain these expectations with regard to sexuality.

Practical steps such as prolonging foreplay, using gels for lubrication and topical estrogens may be of help when the problem resides in sexual response. Systemic estrogen and testosterone have been shown to be effective. Estrogen and testosterone act locally to increase the genital sensitivity, congestion and lubrication and centrally to increase sexual fantasies and sexual desire. Although there is anxiety about testosterone supplements in many women and some medical practitioners, our own extensive experience with testosterone implants shows that after adequate explanation most women with a sexual response disorder will try an implantation at least once. The main points in counseling are summarized in Table 9.12. Recently, testosterone patches have been developed. In controlled studies a 300 µg patch was shown to be safe and effective treatment for sexual dysfunction in women over 48 years of age who had undergone a hysterectomy or oophorectomy. Additional benefits of testosterone are increases in lean body mass and bone density.

Adverse side-effects are uncommon, but oily skin and acne are reported with frequency. The incidence of hirsutism is less than 1% in our clinic. Alopecia, voice change and clitoromegaly are rare, so it is not possible to give an accurate estimate. Altered lipid profile does not represent a real problem. In our opinion, testosterone supplementation is an under-utilized treatment option.

ACKNOWLEDGEMENT

The author would like to thank Dr Fran Reader, Consultant in Reproductive Health Ipswich Hospital, UK who revised the manuscript and made helpful suggestions.

Further reading

Bancroft J. *Human Sexuality and its Problems*. Edinburgh: Churchill Livingstone, 1989

Basson R, Berman J, Burnett A, *et al*. Report of the international consensus development conference of female sexual dysfunction: definitions and classifications. *J Sex Marital Ther* 2001;27:83–94

Diokno A, Brown M, Herzog A. Sexual function in the elderly. *Arch Intern Med* 1990;150:197–200

Griffin M. The sexual health of women after the menopause. *Sex Marital Ther* 1995;10:277–91

Hawton K. *Sex Therapy – A Practical Guide*. Oxford: Oxford Medical Publications, 1985

Lauman E, Paik A, Rosen R. Sexual dysfunction in the United States. *J Am Med Assoc* 1999;281:537–44

Meston C, Frohlich P. The neurobiology of sexual function. *Arch Gen Psychiatry* 2000;57:1012–30

Modelska K, Cummings S. Female sexual dysfunction in postmenopausal women: systematic review of placebo-controlled trials. *Am J Obstet Gynecol* 2003;188:286–93

Osborn M, Hawton K, Gath D. Sexual dysfunction among middle age men in the community. *Br Med J* 1988;296:959–62

Reader F. Female sexual problems. In Studd J, ed. *The Year Book of the Royal College of Obstetricians and Gynaecologists*. London: Royal College of Obstetricians and Gynaecologists Press, 1996: 223–34

Reader F, ed. Minisymposium – psychosexual disorders. *The Diplomate* 1997;4:264–89

Shifren JL, Braunstein GD, Simon JA, *et al*. Transdermal testosterone treatment in women with impaired sexual function after oophorectomy. *N Engl J Med* 2000;343:682–8

Wellings K, Field Y, Johnson A, Wadsworth J. *Sexual Behaviour in Britain*. London: Penguin, 1994

Appendix I

Currently available combined oral contraceptive pills in the UK

Hormone content	Proprietary name	Estrogen dose (μg)	Progestogen dose (μg)
Second-generation pills			
Ethinylestradiol and levonorgestrel	Microgynon 30/Ovranette	30	150
	Eugynon 30/Ovran 30	30	250
	Ovran	50	250
	Trinordiol/Logynon	30/40/30	50/75/125
Ethinylestradiol and norethisterone	Ovysmen/Brevinor	35	500
	Norimin	35	1000
	Binovum	35	500/1000
	Trinovum	35	500/750/1000
	Synphase	35	500/1000/500
Ethinylestradiol and norethisterone acetate	Loestrin 20	20	1000
	Loestrin 30	30	1500
Mestranol and norethisterone	Norinyl-1	50	1000
Third-generation pills			
Ethinylestradiol and desogestrel	Mercilon	20	150
	Marvelon	30	150
Ethinylestradiol and gestodene	Femodene/Minulet	30	75
	Tri-Minulet/Triadene	30/40/30	50/70/100
Ethinylestradiol and norgestimate	Cilest	35	250
Not yet classified			
Ethinylestradiol and drospirenone	Yasmin	30	3

Appendix II

Prevention of pelvic inflammatory disease at the time of IUD insertion

Treat the patient as an individual

(1) Consider all relevant methods of contraception.

(2) Explain the risks of PID to the patient. Tell her why you are going to ask questions about her personal life.

(3) Assess her risk:

    (a) Age;
    (b) Recent change of partner (< six months);
    (c) Genital symptoms or low abdominal/pelvic pain (two or more sexual partners in the last 12 months).

(4) If at risk of an STI consider other methods.

Intrauterine device insertions

(1) **All women** having an IUD inserted should be advised of the risk of pelvic infection after this procedure, taking into account any risk factors for STIs that they might have themselves, e.g., young age (≤ 25 years) or multiple partners. The risks in the absence of an STI are low, being under 1% (as low as 0.1% in 'low-risk' women); however, should PID develop there is a 6% risk of subfertility.

(2) **Nulliparous women under 35 years**: If an IUD is being considered for women in this category, the standard management is to take tests for genital infections (see below) and if they are negative to fit a device. Antibiotic prophylaxis (see below) may also be offered.

(3) **Nulliparous women over 35 years not at risk for sexually transmitted infection**: An antibiotic prophylaxis may be offered.

(4) **Parous women over 35 years at risk of a sexually transmitted infection**: If an IUD is being considered for women in this group, the standard management is to take tests for genital infections (see below) and if they are negative to fit a device.

(5) **Parous women over 35 years in long-term monogamous relationships**: There is no need to offer screening for STIs or antibiotic prophylaxis.

Antibiotic prophylaxis available in family planning clinics

Azithromycin 1 g stat and Metronidazole 400 mg bd. for five days.

What tests should be done?

When testing for STIs the following tests should always be done:

(1) High vaginal swab (charcoal transport medium) for microscopy, culture and sensitivity (MC&S) analysis;

(2) Endocervical swab (charcoal transport medium) for MC&S analysis; and

(3) Endocervical and urethral chlamydia swabs for ligase chain reaction assays.

Index